Making Good On Private Duty

Practical Hints To Graduate Nurses

by

Harriet Camp Lounsbery

Double 9 BOOKS

Making Good On Private Duty
Practical Hints To Graduate Nurses
by Harriet Camp Lounsbery

ISBN: 978-93-62768-69-8

Published by

DOUBLE 9 BOOKS
2/13-B, Ansari Road
Daryaganj, New Delhi – 110002
info@double9books.com
www.double9books.com
Tel. 011-40042856

ABOUT THE AUTHOR

Harriet Camp Lounsbery, an esteemed figure in nursing literature, presents her masterpiece "Making Good On Private Duty: Practical Hints To Graduate Nurses," offering invaluable guidance and insights to aspiring healthcare professionals. Through meticulous attention to detail and a wealth of practical experience, Lounsbery provides a comprehensive resource tailored specifically to graduate nurses, equipping them with the knowledge and skills needed to excel in private duty nursing. In this seminal work, Lounsbery combines her expertise as a nurse educator and practitioner to address the unique challenges and responsibilities faced by graduate nurses entering the field. From patient care techniques to professional etiquette, she offers practical advice and actionable strategies to navigate the complexities of private duty nursing with confidence and competence. With a focus on real-world scenarios and hands-on solutions, "Making Good On Private Duty" serves as an indispensable companion for nurses transitioning from the classroom to the bedside. Lounsbery's dedication to the nursing profession shines through in every page, making this book a timeless resource for generations of nurses seeking to make a meaningful impact in their practice.

CONTENTS

PREFACE

Though technic is constantly changing, methods improving, and the teaching in our schools grows better and more comprehensive, the old problems in private work are ever to be faced, and still the young sister in our nursing world needs to be counselled, guided and helped. It is for these young private duty nurses that this book has been written.

For six years I went up and down one of our large cities doing private nursing, and I can remember, as if it were but yesterday, the curious little sinking of the heart I used to feel, as I mounted the steps of a house where there was a new patient needing my care. "Would I do everything right?" "Could I please the patient and the friends?" "Would the doctor be satisfied with my efforts?" "How would I feel when I was leaving?" "Encouraged or hopeless?" "Happy or sad?" A strange house looks so forbidding, "would this one ever look friendly?" There is time, while walking up the steps, for these and many more such thoughts to crowd into the nurse's mind. Once in the presence of the patient, however, all this quickly changes, and action puts all wondering and doubt to flight.

The "hints" here given are the fruit of my own experience and that of the graduates of the school of which I was the superintendent. Many long talks we had, when they felt the need of coming back to their hospital home for advice and comfort. It is an earnest wish to help the young graduate over the intricate paths that the inexperienced nurse must often tread that has led me to revise some early contributions [Footnote: Printed by permission of the *Trained Nurse*.] to the *Trained Nurse* and write a few new ones, which have within the past year appeared in the *American Journal of Nursing*.

In the chapter "Hints to the Obstetrical Nurse," there is little or nothing that is commonly taught in the class-room.

All of that is so well done, repetition here would be tiresome. All the asepsis is familiar to every graduate. She knows how to sterilize any and every thing, but sometimes she does not know the best way to wash and dry the baby's little shirts or knitted shawls. Sometimes she will not realize that if the layette cannot be purchased at a store, old table linen makes the best diapers for the newborn baby, and that his pillowcase should not have embroidery in the center.

I wish in this part to give the nurse such hints that she may be able to help any woman who wishes to prepare for her confinement. I have been asked so many times to tell a young expectant mother just *what* to get, that I have made for convenience as full a list as is necessary for any baby or mother, with some hints as to the washing of the baby. The rest it is expected every nurse who graduates from a training-school would know. The table for calculating an expectant confinement was cut from a medical paper and given me by a physician some years ago. He did not know who wrote it, nor do I, but he always used it, and I have found it most accurate.

The recipes I have given are, I know, reliable, having all been tested many times. Most of the articles of food every nurse has probably prepared, but exact proportions have a dreadful way of slipping out of one's memory. Whether it is a pint of milk or a quart that must be mixed with two eggs for a custard might not seem much of a problem to a housekeeper, but to a nurse who has perhaps not made a custard for a year it might carry many difficulties.

I have tried to help in this most important part of a nurse's duty, and not only as to the food served the patient, but the *manner* of serving it, which last is truly to a sick person of as much importance as the food itself. The few leaves I have left blank are for such additional recipes as every nurse will gather as she goes from house to house. Any cook will be glad to give some hints as to how she does this or that, and no nurse should be too proud to learn from the cook, or anybody else. I shall never forget the fat little Irish woman who taught me to make clam broth, or how much pride she took in my first success. To ask the family cook for advice is sometimes good policy; she is often so ready to resent any extra work caused by the sickness or the nurse, it pays well to conciliate her, by asking for her aid or counsel. To feel that she can teach the "Trained Nurse" will often make a friend of the cook, and this will make things pleasanter all around. It is with the hope that these homely and perhaps somewhat old-fashioned hints may be of real service, that this little book is sent forth to do what good it may to those who are setting out on their professional careers. It is ever to the young that we elders look, knowing, as Mrs. Isabel Hampton Robb has truly said, "Work shall be lifted from our hands and carried on to loftier ideals and higher aims by the strong young hands, hearts and brains of future nurses." H. C. L.

Charleston, W. Va.

I
THE NURSE AND HER PATIENT

You may think it unnecessary for me to tell you any more about "the patient." You will say, perhaps: "Have I had all this training, and must I yet be told how to treat a patient?" I answer that you have been taught how to watch the progress of disease, how to follow intelligently the doctor's orders, also certain manual arts, your proficiency in which is unquestionably most necessary, but there is much more comprehended in the meaning of the term "a good nurse" than this. How often do we hear stories of nurses who were good—*but*—who were skillful—*but*— and after the *but* comes a long list of such faults as do not show so much in hospital life, where the routine and the many rules and the constant supervision make them less likely to become prominent. "She bangs the doors." "She breaks the fine china." "She wears heavy shoes," or "She talks too much," or "She is pretty and spends too much time over her front hair"—but why go on? You have all heard such tales—*ad nauseam*, and if you are wise, you will set up a sign-post against every one of these snares into which your sister nurses have fallen, and on this you will print in large, clear letters: "Danger! Walking on this place forbidden." So much by way of apology for treating you once more to a lecture on "the patient."

The relation between nurse and patient should, from the first, be a more than amicable one. You have come to bestow the priceless blessing of unwearied, skillful care upon one who should thankfully receive it, and believe me, if you do not go to your patient with a feeling of thankfulness to God for allowing you to assume such a sacred trust as the care of a human life, you are in no condition to undertake the work. Your nursing should be, in a way, an exponent of your own spiritual state; looking at it in its highest aspect, an outward and visible sign of an inward and spiritual grace.

In the first place, then, you must be in entire sympathy with the sick one—and here do not mistake me—by sympathy I do not mean sentimentalism. The two emotions are as far asunder as the poles. Sympathy, then, you must have, and if you do not intuitively feel it, let me tell you what to do to rouse your dormant feelings. Try earnestly to put yourself in the patient's place. Has she had an operation of some kind, and you have all night been trying to keep her quiet on her back, and she has been begging you to let her turn "never so little?" When you go to lie down, and have, perhaps, a backache, and feel tired, instead of settling yourself in the most comfortable position you can, lie straight and square on your back and say to yourself, "Now I can't turn over," and imagine you have by your side a nurse who will not let you turn. You will find out in the course of an hour that your patient has had a good excuse for all her complaints, and the next night you will know just where to slip your hand in the hollow of the back or under the shoulders to give a little ease. The patient will profit by such exercise on the part of the nurse, and your sympathies will be quickened. Never forget that *the patient is sick*, and you are *not*. You can, you must be firm in what you know is for your patient's best good, but you must never be dictatorial or argumentative. It is hard, I know, to bear with all the foolish, unreasonable whims of sick people, but if you are true nurses you will do it. There are, however, several consoling thoughts which have always helped me, and which I will tell you. In the first place, always remember, as I said before, that the sick one *is* sick, and on that ground you can overlook much. In the second place, remember that it will not last long. A few days or weeks will surely bring a change. She cannot, in the nature of disease, remain for long in the very trying stage, unless indeed she have some kind of mania, and of course if that is the case, you need pay no attention to her whims. If she says white is black, let it go. It does not make it so to have her say so, but if you argue the point, and bring all your wisdom to bear upon your demonstration, you may bring her pulse and temperature up to a point that will do her a real injury.

Tact, as you know, is worth everything to you, and by it you will win your way to all hearts. Try then to feel as the patient does, and you will know by instinct how to treat her, and will, perhaps, be often rewarded for some little deed by the pleased surprise with which she will say, "How did you know I wanted it done?" You need not tell her how you knew, but you may be sure she will appreciate you all the more for your prescient thoughtfulness. Her pillows may be flat and hot, her hair uncomfortable, her under sheet wrinkled or untucked from the bottom; all these and a dozen more little things can be arranged so easily, and they conduce so much to the sick one's comfort when done, that you must ever have them in your mind.

Be most careful also as to your patient's belongings, her top drawer, her various boxes, and her linen closet. You must keep all these things just as she did. You may think it a very foolish thing for her to have three piles of handkerchiefs, each of a different age, or degree of fineness, but if that is her way, she will be better satisfied if she knows you will not lay a fine handkerchief over a more common one. So keep them as carefully divided as if they were the two parts of a Seidlitz powder.

Hang her clothes up carefully whenever she goes back to bed, be it once or oftener during the day. Separate them and hang them up; don't pick all up together and put them over a chair. Put her shoes away, lay the stockings on a shelf or put them inside the shoes. Fold her pretty shawl or kimono and lay it in a drawer. Let her see that you know a good thing, and know how to take care of it.

Put away fine china or glass and bric-a-brac, if she is very ill, and you need space for necessary glasses or other articles. It will be a pleasant way of beguiling the tedium of some long day in her convalescence to bring forth and arrange them in their accustomed places. Be careful of books, table-covers, and all the articles of luxury and beauty you will find in many of our city houses. Remember that these things belong to some one else, though you are for the present custodian, and think how provoked you would feel if some stranger should come to your home, and, even if she did nurse you back to health, she left many nicked plates, broken vases and handleless cups behind her. I think you would not want her to nurse you again.

I saw recently in an English magazine devoted to nursing, a very clever article on "Talk." The writer, a nurse, thought subjects were scarce. She says: "We must not talk to the patient about her own complaint, that would make her morbid; or about the doctor, for that would be gossip; or the hospital, for hospitals are full of horrors; or the other nurses, for that might lead to talking scandal; or about other patients, for that would be betrayal of confidence. Now what *are* you to talk about when a patient is well enough to talk, and your talking to her will not hurt her (but on this point be very sure before you air your eloquence)? It is indeed quite a question, and the nurse must often use all her ingenuity to keep the patient to the right subjects, for even patients, though they hold it so reprehensible in a nurse to talk gossip, do not disdain to serve up their neighbors occasionally to the nurse, with some very highly seasoned scandal sauce, and here the honor of the nurse must come into play; let her forget it if possible, as woe will betide the poor girl if in her next place she unwittingly lets out any of the secrets she has heard in these long talks. Try then to steer clear of the neighbors. If your patient be a cultivated person, and you yourself know anything about books, you have a never-failing topic. All the latest books, the famous books, the most entertaining books, and if you can read aloud and the patient likes to hear you, read to her, and it will do both good—only be sure not to tire her by reading too much at one time. Talk of interesting places you have visited and she will do the same, of pictures you have seen, and last, but not least, you can talk about clothes. Generally the first serious piece of business a convalescent concerns herself about is the purchase and making of some new clothes. She wants something new and fresh, and if you can give her any new ideas on the subject or tell her of any pretty materials you have seen in the shop windows, you will prove as entertaining as if you talked on any of the forbidden topics, and many times more useful."

I would like, in closing this chapter, to say a word as to reading the daily papers. If your patient is a woman, she will want to know just about what you, yourself, would be interested in, and this is very easy; but if your patient is a man, it is harder to know what he will want; politics, the money market, etc., which most women skip over. If then your patient is a man, commence on the first page and read slowly the headings of the news items, when one strikes him, as desirable to hear, he will tell you to read it; when you get through the news you may turn to the editorial page and do the same there. Unless you know your patient very well do not attempt to enlighten him as to the stock market quotations, for it is, I suppose, well nigh impossible for an ordinary woman to read them so that a man will understand her. He will probably laugh over your well meant endeavor, and ask you to "kindly let him look at the paper," when he will in a moment find out what you have been trying to say.

II
THE NURSE AND THE DOCTOR

I suppose no nurse goes through a training school without being duly impressed by all the doctors on the staff of lecturers that they, the doctors, are the generals of the campaign. She and her fellows are the aids, and that she will be kind enough to remember this fact, and not make suggestions to him, the doctor, or give him the fruits of her ripe experience of three years in a hospital, and more or less time, as may be, since she has graduated. But though this I think you all know, there are some points of your connections with the doctor which may not be quite so clear.

In the first place, then, remember that you are his *aid,* you are to help him in every way you can, you are never to work against him, never weaken the patient's confidence in him. If you do not understand why he does thus and so, ask for an explanation, if you know him pretty well, and if your questions are reasonable ones, and intelligently put, he will be glad to answer you, and explain all you wish explained; but if you do not know the reason of a certain order, and, moreover, if he will not tell you, do not assume that he does not know, or that he is cross; it may be some very uncertain, delicate experiment is being tried, and all he wants you to do is to tell him, with a free unbiased mind, what you see. Always, however, be loyal to him with the patient. When you are asked a thousand questions as to, "Why doesn't the doctor do this, or why does he do that?" you can always say that he does it, or does it not, for the patient's best good, of that you are assured, and they must be also.

You collect the facts and put them in an orderly way before the doctor; upon your observations and reports he bases his theories of the disease in many cases. You can see what perfect faith he must have in you, and how true you must be to him in order to secure your patient's best good. I have often heard doctors say, when speaking of a favorite nurse, as if it was the only virtue worth mentioning: "I am perfectly certain that when I am not present she will *faithfully* carry out my orders." Entire faithfulness takes precedence, I think, and deservedly so. Your accomplishments may be many, but if you have not this faithfulness, this obedience to the doctor as a rudder to the ship of your professional character, no matter how great may be the load of learning and accomplishments and good intentions, your self-will and vanity will bring you to the rocks where ruin is inevitable.

Do not fear losing your own individuality and independence. "He who obeys well, governs well," is a very old, and a very true saying, and your responsibilities will never cease. The more faithful you are to orders, the more trust and confidence will be reposed in you. You will have not only your patient, but the entire family looking to you for directions, for, upon your faithfulness, and the tact with which you administer your authority, will depend much of your success as nurses.

Be careful not to sever your relations with any patient unless your doctor knows all about it. Never leave your charge, no matter how urgent the reason may be, unless you tell him. You may be sick, or the place may be unsuited to you, or you to the place, and you may know that it is best for you to go. But speak first to the doctor, tell him candidly why you wish to go, and take counsel of him how you should act. If he tells you you may go, and you know that your place must be filled, do not offer as your substitute your best friend, or anyone else. If he wishes your counsel he will ask, and then you may tell him of anyone you think will suit the position, but do not offer your friend, as he may have some favorite of his own to put in your place. Of course the patient or her friends must know about the contemplated change— that I take for granted. Having consulted the doctor, will make everything satisfactory to the most careful practitioner. So, as said before, never go away from your patient, leaving in your place a nurse whom the doctor does not know. He has, in most cases, selected you for his patient, and he wants you, you may not be all he wishes you were, but still such as you are, *there* you are, he knows what you can and what you cannot do; and it is a great piece of impertinence for a nurse to go away unknown to the doctor, leaving a stranger in her place. The consequence, so far as he is concerned, will most likely be to have her name crossed off his list as "unreliable"—so be careful.

As to your records, keep them faithfully; the doctor usually looks them over very carefully, but sometimes you find one who passes them over in a lofty manner, rather trying when you take such pains with them. You may conclude that it is not necessary to keep them accurately in such a case, but this same doctor may ask you some day how long ago it was that the patient's temperature took such a sudden rise, or how many days it is since she first had solid food, and if you have accurately kept and carefully preserved your records, you can tell without a moment's hesitation. It is better, more business-like, and every way to be commended, that the nurse should keep, and be exceedingly particular about these records. If the doctor will write his orders on the fresh daily record at his morning visit, it is a great help to the nurse, but very often he is in a hurry and you must write them yourself. If you have to do this, take your record and write as he tells you, *when* he tells you. If the orders are at all intricate it is your only way of being absolutely sure you have everything correct. It is a protection to you also, if the family are inclined to criticise.

A nice little point for you to remember is always to leave the doctor *alone* with the patient for a few moments, if it is at all possible, at each visit, Wait until he has asked all the questions he wishes, or until you have told him all that is necessary to tell before the patient, and then on some errand, real or imaginary, leave the room. Of course, if the patient is desperately ill, you cannot do this, nor will it then be necessary.

It is a good plan to wait for the doctor at the head of the stairs, or at the foot, if you are likely to be over-heard, and tell him there all you could not say before the patient as to her condition, etc. He likewise may have something to say,—some final instruction to give, some caution he would not wish the patient to know of. This is also the time to speak about yourself if you are sick or tired, or unhappy in your position. Perhaps neither of you have anything to say, and a friendly nod and a "patient is doing nicely, nurse," will send you back to the sick- room feeling that your work is appreciated, which always goes a long way toward making the hard places easy. Your patients may be very curious as to what you have to say to the doctor, but you can readily and truly tell them that there are many things you have to say to him, that would be hard for you to say before them, and hard for them to hear too, and these are things you arrange outside.

Always be sure to have on a convenient table, if your doctor be of a homoeopathic school, a little covered tray, and on it two glasses, clean, and turned upside down to keep them from dust, teaspoons and covers for the glasses, also a small pitcher of fresh water. Many doctors of the old school also use some medicines in water, so it is best to have glasses always at hand.

Do not sit down when the doctor is making his professional call, unless he or the patient requests it. He will probably sit at the side of the bed, your place is at or near the foot. If the doctor knows the patient well, as a friend, and is inclined to stay a long time, chatting, you can go quietly to another part of the room, and take up your work or reading, but be sure the doctor has finished asking you questions before you go.

Use sparingly technical terms. If your patient's feet are oedematous, tell the doctor they are much swollen; if he *ask* if they are oedematous tell him "yes," but do not volunteer to name the peculiar kind of swelling. If the abdomen is tympanitic, tell him it seems much distended; and if he questions much further, answer the questions fully and intelligently. If your patient has the symptoms of phlebitis, tell him of the rise of temperature, the swelling of the leg, the tenderness along the course of the vein, and he will know that you know and appreciate the gravity of the disease; but be sure you do not attempt to give the symptoms a name, that is not your place.

I would have you be very careful as to what instruments you carry; have them of the best. Let your thermometer be of the very best make.

There is nothing more trying in a small way than to have your thermometer doubted, and if you *know* it is the best the market affords, if you take it to the instrument maker and have it tested once in a while, you need not fear, when you find an unusual temperature, and report it to the doctor, and he quietly proceeds to test your thermometer by his, which of course is always correct. Be sure that your hypodermic syringe will work; if the piston slips loosely after much using of brandy, aromatic ammonia, etc., take it to be repaired, and see that the needles are sharp, they become dulled very quickly; keep also the tiny wires pushed through them. It is just as well to keep this syringe in the room, its little case is very small and unobtrusive, and if you keep it near your thermometer in some safe, handy place, you will have it when some unforeseen emergency arises, and you do not want to lose time going to your room for it.

III
THE NURSE HERSELF

It is just as necessary for the nurse to be careful of herself as of the patient, though her care must be manifested in a far different way. Always remember that to do really good work you must have really good tools. No man owning, and intelligently working a valuable machine, would keep it going at its highest speed all the time. He takes care of it, keeps it clean, renews defective parts, oils it; and then he expects it to run for so many hours, and to run well,—to do its work thoroughly. But with all his keeping it in order he does not make it work night and day for weeks or months. Such folly is never heard of in an engineer; but with us human beings, who own and manage a far more wonderful machine than any steam engine, we hear of it often, and always, *always* the tale winds up with the inevitable catastrophe. The business man develops paresis, the clergyman loses his voice or his eyes, the nurse contracts some disease that incapacitates her for work, in every case mother Nature makes the careless or ignorant owner of the wonderful machine pay the penalty of the misuse. It does not matter to Nature what the reason is for our breaking the great laws; we can kill ourselves with philanthropic work just as surely as with over indulgence. One trouble is, that it does not always *kill*. A paralytic may live for years, so does a man with paresis. When the wonderful God-given machine works badly, or stops entirely, we look on, and sometimes wonder why it is that those who are so helpful, such fine examples of courage, of skill, of virtue, so hardly to be spared, are the ones to be taken away. Do *we* wonder, we who are nurses? Do we not know what did it? Ah! yes—we know, we know, that such and such a nurse was tired out when she went to still another case—and when we heard she herself was ill we were not slow to say, "Foolish girl! Did she suppose she was made of wrought iron and sole leather?" But will *we* take heed, and not do likewise, or will we wonder, with the unthinking ones, why it is that the good, useful people are always taken away? Do not deceive yourselves; they are not "taken away," they take themselves away, for God will not reverse His wise laws because we (no matter how good we are) act in defiance of them.

Please remember I am only speaking now to the good nurses—the enthusiastic ones,—poor nurses, lazy nurses have no temptation to overwork themselves. They may die of indigestion, but they will not die of exhaustion.

It seems to you so natural for others to be sick. You have seen the sick by scores in the hospital, and have waited on them, felt sorry for them, sympathized with them; but have you thought that it was within the bounds of possibility that *you* could ever come into such a pitiable condition? You go from house to house in your private nursing, always you find the sick, and it seems natural, quite the proper thing. You care for them, they get well, or die—and on you go to the next—but reflect on what made them sick, and though you *know* you are made of like flesh and blood, do not conduct yourself as if you were not. "Oh, yes" (how often have I heard it said), "I know she worked too hard, but I am so strong, you never heard *me* complain; I can nurse a fever case for two weeks and never go out of doors for air or exercise." Is it not foolish? Is it not wrong for any sensible woman to talk thus?

Now listen to some few practical hints as to how to keep yourselves in good working order. In the first place, then, never go to a case unless you are feeling well. It is far wiser, as far as you are concerned, and better also for the sick one, for you to say so frankly, if you are not well. Tell the one who comes for you, that you could not do justice to the case, as indeed you could not. Sick people are as sensitive as babies to the subtle influence exerted by the one who is so constantly over them. If you are in full health and strength, your rubbing will be quieting and effectual, your very presence, if you are careful and gentle, will be soothing. On the contrary, if you yourself are suffering and are using the nervous force you ought to be giving your patient in hiding your own malady, your presence will not be so eagerly welcomed; your patient will not know what is the matter, but she feels rather a relief when you are absent. Going to a case feeling perfectly well, the next thing is to keep well.

Be careful about your *eating*. Your meals will of necessity be often irregular, that is unavoidable, but eat only wholesome things. Do not eat candy; and at dinner, which you will probably have in the evening after the family are through, avoid patties, and rich puddings, ice cream, and such like. You will always find plenty of plain food and fruit in the most luxurious homes; eat these and let the rest alone. If you want to keep your stomach and whole digestive apparatus in good order, you must care for it, and not overtax it. If you have a pretty good stomach it will bear a good deal of abuse, but in the end it will grumble, and a dyspeptic nurse is not an attractive object. As to your night suppers, which you should always have, should your case require constant watching, I would recommend plenty of coffee, tea, or cold milk, if you can drink it, bread and butter, cold meat and fruit. Never eat candied fruits, cake, or pies at night. Have eggs if you care for them, and pickles if you like. Remember, the plainest food, the most easily digested, the most nourishing is what you must have. Believe me, you will be rewarded for the temperate use you make of all the dainties you see, by a clear complexion, and good color, which will make you "good to look at," especially good for a sick person to look at.

As to the nurse's night toilette, it is quite a problem sometimes as to just what is best to wear. When the patient is not ill enough for the uniform to be retained for night duty, the nurse should be comfortable enough so that she can sleep; yet dressed enough for any emergency. I think a house gown of pretty material much neater than the kimono. Be sure this fits about the shoulders, and never have loose flowing sleeves. A white frill in the neck looks very trim, and is always becoming. The corset and all tight clothes should be removed, stockings and underwear kept on. The hair should be arranged simply, but not allowed to hang in a loose braid, unless you are *very* sure you will not see any but the patient, and even then it may be unwise, as a braid of hair has an exasperating way of slipping from its proper place (hanging down the back) and dipping into whatever you are stooping over. Dressed thus, with night shoes to protect the feet, one can lie down on a lounge and sleep very comfortably, being freed from tight clothes, and yet being entirely presentable, no matter what happens. To undress regularly and put on the diaphanous low-necked short sleeved night dress of the present mode, and go to bed, when you are sure you will have to get up one or a dozen times during the night is not good judgment, I think. You get out of a warm bed, and if you only put on your shoes and stockings, your patient must wait while you do it. If anything serious occurs suddenly, you either run the risk of taking cold from being insufficiently clad while doing what must be done, or your patient must wait while you dress—both bad.

Never get into bed with your patient. This seems to most people a quite unnecessary caution, but it is the commonest experience of the successful nurse, that a woman, feeble and nervous, should ask and almost insist that she shall lie down by her, or get into bed with her. I always wonder that a sick woman can not realize that she is not a pleasant bed-fellow, but she seldom does. Of course you are not to tell her that she is not fit to sleep with, but you *can* say that she needs and ought to have the whole bed to herself, and you will sit by her and hold her hand, or if she insists on it, you can lie down, with your house gown on, on the *outside* of the bed, being careful to give her plenty of space, and when she is asleep, get up quietly and lie down on your lounge, which should be placed so that you can see her every movement.

Never let the patient think for a moment that you fear her disease; if she has diphtheria, do not tell her or the family that you have a delicate throat or that it is sore, and do not examine it by the help of a hand-glass where any one can see you. Do not go to such cases if you really fear them, but if you go, and have reason to feel that you have contracted the disease, tell the doctor as soon as you can, and if he thinks you ill, he will send you home. Never tell a patient you have a weak back or any weakness. Tell the doctor and he will see to it that you have rest or medicine, but do not let the patient know it. Never go about a sick room with a long face; it is enough for the sick one to have to be sick; the family sympathies are all enlisted for her. You are there to be a help and a comfort, not an added anxiety. Of course these remarks do not apply to any of you who are tired from a long, exhausting case. The family in such instances are ready and willing enough to let you rest. Keep your cheery manner: all higher considerations aside, it is money in your pocket to look cheerful. I have known one or two good, faithful, conscientious nurses who were dismissed from case after case, merely because they looked "so doleful." It may seem curious to place a commercial value on a smile, but in reality it amounts almost to that.

Be very careful to have your dresses fit you perfectly, and have them well laundered, especially do not have them too stiff. In this connection I cannot do better than to relate an incident that I heard of some time ago. A nurse went to care for a patient whose first nurse had been called to her own home, and she had not been in the room an hour before the patient called her and taking her hand said, "My dear, I can't tell you how thankful I feel that your dress is not too short in the waist. Miss——'s dress was frightful!" This was only a nervous woman's whim, but our success as nurses depends in many cases on just such whims, so it is well to be careful. When the patient is well enough for you to come to the family table at meal time, be sure to have on a spotless apron, and let no sickroom odors announce your presence. It is worth more to a nurse to have soft, dry, warm, sympathetic hands, than to have the prettiest face ever seen under a cap, so be careful of them; after using any antiseptics always have at hand glycerin and rose water, cold cream, or something soothing to use. Never put a cold or clammy hand on a patient. If it is cold and dry it can be laid on a hot, aching head, but never do so if it is the least damp. If the hand is always damp, pour on it a little alcohol, or eau de cologne, if that is preferred, or some toilet water, then put it on the patient's head, and it will be all right. A simple and very cold lotion is alcohol and water, about equal parts, and a piece of ice added. Hold your hand in this a moment and then gently comb the patient's hair (that which grows on top of the head) with the dripping fingers, taking care not to let any cold water-drops fall on the face. This is wandering somewhat from my subject, but I will let it stand and speak of one more thing that is good to remember. Never lay a warm hand on a patient's head, or a cold one on the body. If you have to rub your patient's body, and your hand is warm and damp, shake a little talcum powder into it, or use a little cold cream, cocoa butter, or lanolin, and the dampness will not be perceived. Alcohol may also be used, or bay rum.

Some nurses are much troubled by excessive perspiration, especially under the arms, any hard work making the dress quite wet. The ordinary shields are not very good, as they are not absorbent enough. A piece of flannel basted inside of the shield is a help, as that is absorbent. The auxiliary space might be bathed with a solution of alum; alcohol is good or alcohol with white-oak bark. Many preparations for this trouble are on the market, most of them are good but some are expensive. A late copy of the *Journal of Nursing* gives the following: "Take two ounces of baking soda, mix with half an ounce of corn starch, and use as a dusting powder, after the parts have been thoroughly cleansed and dried. It will check the perspiration and remove every particle of odor." This is very successful, but I find it leaves a slight yellow stain on a white dress. Another remedy from *Journal of Nursing* is this: "Zinc oxide" applied to axillae twice a week, after bathing at night, will dissipate the odor. If the perspiration has a disagreeable odor, no effort should be spared to free oneself from what is a serious drawback to the acceptableness of a nurse.

Be very careful not to contract any little annoying habits, such as frequent clearing of the throat, sniffing, etc. You may have a catarrh, but use your handkerchief quietly; such noises are very disgusting, and these habits, I am sorry to say, are not rare, and seem very hard to conquer.

I suppose that I have better opportunities to hear stories of nurses and their doings, good and evil, than some have. I certainly hear some very curious things. The most extraordinary was of a nurse who always made it a rule, when she went to a patient's house, to stipulate immediately for her hours "off duty." She thought she was doing a very clever thing, and making a most commendable business-like arrangement. It will not be necessary for me to show you what a lack of tact she exhibited, and what an antagonistic feeling she aroused.

Never kiss your patient or allow yourself to show any demonstrative affection, unless you are very sure it will be welcome, and be careful even then. A kiss for "goodbye" when you leave the patient is usually quite enough, and many ladies are repulsed by anything of the kind. If you feel an affectionate regard for your patient, you can show it by your constant thoughtfulness and your care. Do not fear that you will lead lonesome, repressed lives; if you are the nurses you ought to be, you will have all the affection you want, and often more than you know what to do with. Never do any sewing or fancy work for yourself until you are sure there is none you could do for the patient. Remember that she pays for your time, and govern yourself accordingly.

Read to her, sew for her, play cards with her, but do not amuse yourself or regulate your wardrobe at her expense. When I say "sew for her" I do not mean make her dresses, but do the little odd things that mothers of families always do, and which must remain undone if she is sick, unless you do them. Do not write letters when on duty, and, above all things, do not write with a scratchy pen. To a nervous person the sound of a scratchy pen traveling over the paper is torturing, and it can be heard even if you are in the next room. A fountain pen is, I think, the best to use. See that it is full before you go to your case, and it will need no attention for three or four weeks. This pen makes no noise as you write, and you have it always at hand, and if you have to leave your letter in haste, you can put the cap on the pen and slip it in your pocket, and no one is in any danger of finding fault with the nurse for leaving an open ink-bottle for somebody to tip over.

Remember finally (and I think, from what I read in the daily papers, you are in no danger of forgetting this), that you are not domestics, and, while in an emergency I would have you shrink from nothing that needs doing, I do not think you should do any washing. Cooking you will very often have to do, but the ordinary housework does not come at all into your province. If your patient is a chronic invalid, I would have you make yourself useful in the house. Do the shopping, order the meals, anything that will show your patient you are anxious to help make the wheels of domestic machinery run more smoothly.

You must use all the tact you possess; you will not find two houses just alike, or two patients with the same tastes. A "lady" in an emergency does many things she usually leaves to the servants. So must you. There is sickness, trouble with the servants, every domestic wheel turning with difficulty, and, if you have time, if you can leave your patient without doing her an injury, you can, perhaps, by some little service earn much gratitude from the family, and help to remove the impression that trained nurses are "so helpless and need so much waiting on."

In conclusion, let me tell you, with all the earnestness of which I am capable, that upon each one of you rests not only the reputation of your school, but, in a measure, the reputation of the profession. No one needs to be told how much more widely known is an inconsistent Christian than a faithful one, how much harm one does and how comparatively little good comes of the others' faithfulness. And it is just so with you nurses, a careless nurse makes a far wider reputation than a careful one.

If one physician is unskillful or unprincipled, the whole profession is not found fault with, but the individual is blamed and another one found who will do better, but it is not so in most cases where a nurse proves unsatisfactory. The whole profession suffers and every nurse sinks more or less if one of her sister nurses commits an indiscretion, or does any of the thousand things she ought not to do. I recollect very well, many years ago, a Brooklyn nurse, of about thirty-five years, married her patient, a boy nineteen years old. It made a great stir in the city, and, as I was living there at the time and the superintendent of a training school, I had to bear my share of the odium cast upon all nurses. For months after, almost every one I met took pains to tell me that hereafter they would keep their young sons out of the clutches of the designing nurse, and I doubt not, such slighting remarks were borne by every nurse in town, and it was not pleasant, to say the least of it, for any of us.

Keep your standards high. Let nothing but the very best satisfy you, as far as you and your work are concerned. Keep your mind well informed; if it is full of scientific facts, of skillful methods, of good literature, or fine pictures, there will be no room in it for the memory of all the disagreeable things every one must encounter in one's work, and if you do not remember them, you cannot tell others of them.

Finally, remember (and this lies at the root of it all) to keep your hearts right,—ever thankful that you are permitted to pursue this high calling, and ever striving to be more worthy of it, with many prayers that your life and conduct may show, what is better *lived* than talked about, the grace and peace of God, which verily do pass man's understanding.

IV
THE NURSE AND HER PATIENT'S FAMILY, FRIENDS, AND SERVANTS

Try to realize when you go to a house where there is dangerous illness, that the family is glad to see you when you come. You have come to help them, to stay with them, to comfort them by your presence, by your knowledge, by your experience. They have needed you, have sent for you, and are to pay you for your time. There is a general sense of relief when you are once fairly installed in your place by the bedside, yet you are a stranger. Your friend, the doctor, has told them what a treasure you are. Mrs. This and Mr. That have perhaps let them know how invaluable you were when at their houses; but yet they must look at you a little, they must note if you make a pleasant impression on the invalid, if you are as skillful here as you were somewhere else, if you look with scorn on the plain furniture, or how much you will be displeased that the bath-room is at the other end of the house. They do not feel exactly critical: they are too tired or too anxious for that; but still, unless everyone is too exhausted from watching to do anything but thankfully surrender everything to you, you will be pretty closely looked after at first.

You must look for some espionage; and it is only right that you should be subjected to it. If *your* mother was lying very sick, and some stranger, having knowledge and strength superior to your own, had to come and care for her, would you not feel that though you were glad to see her, glad she would give your mother the benefit of her superior skill, yet you would wish to consider her a little, to note when she did thus and so; or if she did something you did not understand, could you refrain from asking her why she did it?

Be patient, therefore, with the suggestions of the family, after all, though you know the disease and the probable course it will run, the chances for recovery, and what to do in emergency, etc., *they* know the patient, all her peculiarities, her likes and dislikes, and if you are wise you will get and keep many little hints from those who have cared for her before you came. If she likes milk, will she insist upon tea? Does coffee keep her awake? Does she hate the sight of gruel, or beef-tea? Does she like much sugar in her drinks? All these are little matters of individual taste that you must find out for each patient, and if you have the necessary tact and forethought, you never need ask the patient one question; usually the friends are pleased to be consulted on such small matters, and gladly tell you all you wish to know. To be sure, they generally tell much more than you asked for; but that does not matter, it is better to listen patiently for five minutes to someone's tiresome descriptions than to repulse them, and so lose just so much kindly feeling from the one who wished to talk to you.

If the amateur nurse has been doing something actually wrong for the patient, do not tell her so. She did the best she knew how; but say, as pleasantly as you can, "I think perhaps *this* would make our patient more comfortable," or "The doctor thinks such and such things are not now necessary, and it would be better to do this way." Then you can do what you know to be right, and not hurt the feelings of the one who has preceded you, and, feeling your way carefully, have everything just as it ought to be, and no one's feelings will be hurt, and no one will feel that you are looking down upon their ignorance; and here I would say that in your little confidential talks with the doctor, you could ask him to say a word to the family if they persist in doing what you know to be wrong. Ask him to give you orders before some of them, and that will set *you* straight in a moment.

With tact, that most invaluable gift, you can get on with *almost* every one, and when you find that there is no such thing as making friends with the family, you can tell the doctor, and he will let you go; but such places are very rare. Let all see that you are thoroughly interested in your patient, and do not hesitate to perform any little kindness that falls in your way for the rest of the family, and you will win all their hearts without a struggle.

When you go for your rest, be sure to leave carefully written directions for the one who is to take your place, just as you do when in charge of a hospital ward, you leave your orders written out when you go for your "off duty." Show her how to keep the sick-room record, and be sure she understands it all before you leave.

As for the visitors, they are often difficult to manage, and here again you must have the family help you. Of course *no* visitors are allowed until the doctor gives permission. So far all is easy, but when they are admitted you will do well to make a little plan with the family. Tell them the patient may be seen at such an hour. Perhaps between eleven and twelve, perhaps between two and three, just as you consider her brighter in the morning or afternoon. Ask them who of the first and dearest friends is the quietest and most discreet, and then say that if they will kindly arrange for one visitor only to come each day, it would be so much better for the convalescent. The friends can always do this and they never object. They tell Mrs. Jones to come on Monday at two, and stay just fifteen minutes. On Tuesday Mrs. Smith can come, and so on, until by the end of the week the arrangement ceases to cause any comment, and soon, if all goes well, and the convalescence goes on without interruption, *your* rules and extreme care can be relaxed to suit the patient's own fancy.

Always carefully note if any visitor tires your patient, and manage so as not to let her come again until the sick one has more strength. It is better, I think, to sit in an adjoining room when your patient has a visitor. This gives you a chance to come into the room when the person has stayed long enough, and generally your entrance tells her very plainly that she ought to go, and she departs without you saying a word. If she does not, you will have to tell her that the doctor is very particular about not letting the patient talk too much, etc., etc., and get her out in that way. Be careful, when the visitor has gone, not to sit down and talk at length yourself. Give the patient a little nourishment, turn over her pillows, and if she seems at all wearied make her comfortable for a nap and let her sleep.

As to the servants they require pretty careful handling. Above all things, keep on the right side of the *cook*. If you have to go to the kitchen to do any of the cooking, do not make a *mess*, or, if you do, don't run off upstairs and leave it. Gather up your utensils and put them into the sink, and let the water run over them, and ask for the dishcloth: and if you do it pleasantly, the cook will probably tell you to "Niver need thim things," and you will thankfully obey her. If you really cannot stop to make all tidy after your cooking, you can say, "I'm sorry to make you extra work with these dishes, but I must hurry back upstairs." Some such little speech, with a pleasant smile, will make all things easy for you below stairs, and for the sake of all the friction it will save you, it is well worth the trouble. Often the cook will be glad to do the cooking if you tell her how; be careful to tell her, if it is eaten and enjoyed; and never let her know if it is rejected. Get rid of it upstairs by some contrivance, and be sure not to order that dish again. In many cases of course the cook will know all the little dishes the sick one will fancy, and you will have very little to do with her. Such instances are somewhat rare, and very delightful when they occur.

If there is much extra washing, you may have to use much diplomacy as regards the laundress; and if it is very disgusting washing, it is well to have a large pail, with a cover, upstairs. Thoroughly disinfect the clothes before you send them to the washing, as the odors are often sickening, and the laundress, like other servants, is very much afraid, usually, of clothing from a sick-bed. Carry or send the clothes to the washing as soon as possible after removing them from the bed; never, on any account, allow them to remain in the room.

The nurse cannot be too careful as to the amount of clothes she sends to the laundry. She should of course keep herself and the patient scrupulously clean; but she must reflect that private families do not have an unlimited store of towels and sheets, and if she is extravagant in this matter it will seriously detract from her acceptability.

In concluding, let me remind you that all these hints are intended for nurses going from one strange place to another, as you would in nursing fevers, or short surgical cases. Nurses who have chronic cases need none of these rules. They fall into a routine, and if they are detained in the family for any length of time, that shows that their work and methods are right, as far as that patient and family are concerned. But let them be careful when at last they leave the case, and go amongst strangers. The ways of one family are not the ways of another, and they must exercise much discretion to accommodate themselves to the new environment.

V
GENERAL REMARKS ON FOODS AND FEEDING

Always have all food presented to an invalid as tempting as possible. Use pretty china and glass, if you are permitted to do so, yet not the very finest the house affords; that might make the patient nervous lest some evil befall it. Absolutely clean napkins and tray cloths, a few green leaves about the plate, a rose on the tray; the chop or piece of chicken, the bird or the piece of steak ornamented with sprigs of parsley, the cold things really cold, and the hot ones *hot*, these are necessities of invalid's feeding, that mark the nurse who has a proper appreciation of a sick person's delicate sensibilities. Have all plates, cups and saucers *hot*, when they are for the reception of hot toast, coffee, tea, etc. Hot water plates are very convenient, and easily procured at any large china shop; but if they cannot be found, put the hot plate containing the chop over a bowl of boiling water, and cover with a hot saucer, fold a napkin around the baked potato, and you can carry the tray containing the dinner through cold halls and up staircases and it will arrive at your patient's room *hot*. Be careful not to fill the bowl so full of hot water that it will spill. Never fill a cup so full that it will spill its contents over into the saucer, it makes a disgusting looking *mess*. Have all fruit *cold*, oranges and grapes especially. Always look over a bunch of grapes and cut off the soft ones before you hand them to a patient. If you have foreign or California grapes, hold them for a moment under the cold water faucet and let the water run through the bunch, and all the cork dust will then be washed out.

If you peel and quarter an orange for your patient never let her see you do it, unless you are perfectly sure you will not get your hands covered with juice. Wash your hands before you bring it to be eaten.

Be careful not to have any suspicion of grease about the beef tea, broths, etc. A quick and easy way to remove all grease, is to fill a cup or bowl *brimming* full, let it stand a few moments that the grease may rise to the top, tip the cup a very little to one side, and the grease, to the last atom, will flow over the side of the cup; pour your broth carefully into a clean hot cup, and serve. Beef juice is more palatable with a little very brown toast.

Remember, that an invalid hardly ever likes any food made sweet. No matter what the taste may be in health, in sickness, sweet things are nauseous; for this reason ice cream bought at confectioners' is often rejected. Salt also must be used with caution, if the mouth and lips are tender, as is often the case; use the salt sparingly in all broths, etc.

If your patient cannot take milk, when, as in typhoid fever, the doctor wishes the diet to be wholly or for the most part of milk, try at first to remove the thick, bad taste by giving a little pure water or carbonic acid water after it. If that will not do, mix the carbonic acid water with it, and have both nice and cold. If a glass of milk is too much (and it will be in nine cases out of ten, especially if it is cold), give half a glass; if that is still too much, give quarter of a glass, or put more water with it. Never repeat a dose (of food) if it nauseates the patient. Make some change in quantity or quality, and you will, if you watch carefully, find out the right proportions.

A person lying flat down in bed cannot, of course, drink from a glass or cup, and a feeding cup is apt, by pouring too freely, to cause choking. A bent glass tube is the best arrangement, the patient can drink easily through this, and can regulate by sucking, the rapidity with which the food is taken. The tube should be cleaned immediately after each using, and if any beef tea or other food cannot be dislodged by letting water run through it, pass a string with a knot tied in it, through. Make the knot big enough to touch all sides of the tube, have it thoroughly wet, and the cleansing will be easily and quickly accomplished. If a patient prefers drinking from a glass, and can be raised in bed, always lay a napkin under the chin before you give the drink, and on no account have the glass or cup more than half full, if you do, it will surely spill.

In giving medicine that tastes very bitter or unpleasant in any way, bring, at the *same time* with the medicine, some water, milk, or whatever may be preferred, to take after it. Also a napkin to wipe the lips, especially if the patient be a man.

Always keep milk, beef tea, etc., *covered* in the refrigerator, and, if you can, see that this is cleaned every day. But this might cause the cook to feel aggrieved, so I put it as a suggestion merely. But if the refrigerator has a *smell,* and the cook seems touchy, the milk, etc., better be kept upstairs on some sheltered window-ledge, and carefully covered.

If you have your own little refrigerator upstairs, see to it that it is cleaned *every* day. Never put away anything in tin pails; always use earthen or china bowls or pitchers.

BEEF TEA

Beef from the round, finely chopped and free from fat. Proportions, 1 lb. beef to 1 pint of water, cold. Let the beef soak in the water, stirring occasionally, for two hours; then put it on the stove and heat it until the red color disappears; never boil it. Skim off all grease, salt to taste.

BEEF JUICE

Round steak cut an inch thick; slightly broil like beefsteak for the table, cut into squares of an inch, squeeze in a lemon squeezer, skim carefully and salt. Serve either very cold, or place the cup containing the juice in a bowl of boiling water, stir carefully, and as soon as the juice is warm serve. If left a moment too long it is spoiled, as it curdles. One pound of beef makes an after dinner coffee cup almost full of juice.

BEEF TEA IN A BOTTLE

Put into a Mason's preserve jar, tightly corked, one pound of beef chopped as for ordinary beef tea. Put this into a kettle of cold water, with a saucer on the bottom, let it come slowly to a boil and boil for an hour. Take out of the bottle and squeeze the beef.

SCRAPED BEEF

Take a piece of lean round steak, scrape with the edge of a spoon until the place scraped has no more meat on the surface, but only the white fibre, cut this off with a sharp knife, exposing once more a fresh surface. Season, and spread raw on bread and butter, or make into little cakes and broil slightly, according to the doctor's orders, or your patient's taste.

MUTTON BROTH

Mutton from the neck. Proportions, 1 lb. of mutton to 1 quart of water, put the mutton and the water (cold) on the back of the stove, let it come slowly to a boil, boil until the meat is ready to fall from the bones. After straining out all the meat etc. add one tablespoonful of rice or barley. Simmer half an hour after adding rice or barley.

CLAM BROTH. NO. 1

Take 1 qt. clams. Strain off the juice and chop the clams fine, return clams to the juice and simmer one hour. Put on to scald as much milk as juice. Strain out the clams, thicken with a little corn starch, making about as thick as cream, pour juice into a bowl and add the milk.

CLAM BROTH. NO. 2

Same as above, only cut off the hard part of the clams, chop the soft parts and leave them in the broth. For convalescents.

CLAM BROTH. NO. 3

Take little neck clams unopened, wash them very clean with a brush. Place them on the top of the stove in a clean dry pan, and when the shells open take them off, remove the clams and pour the juice into a cup. To be served hot. If it is too strong, add a little boiling water. This is for very sick people; give only a teaspoonful at a time. It sometimes corrects nausea.

CHICKEN BROTH

A fowl, not too young, cut in pieces, 1 qt. water to 1 lb. fowl. Put it on the stove in cold water, let it heat slowly, then boil gently until the meat is ready to fall from the bones, strain, skim and add rice, boil once more for 1/2 hour. Salt to taste. Serve with toast or hot crackers.

OYSTER BROTH

Equal quantities of juice and milk, put each in separate vessels on the stove; when the juice comes to the boil, skim and slightly thicken, pour in the milk boiling hot, add the oysters one by one, let them remain on the stove about five minutes, or until the beards begin to curl, and they are no longer slippery. Serve with crackers heated very hot.

OYSTERS BROILED

Dry the oysters, large ones are best, in a towel, have a piece of toast slightly buttered on a hot plate, near, pour over this a little hot oyster juice, not enough to make the toast wet through. Arrange the oysters on a fine buttered broiler, cook over a brisk fire like steak, until the beards curl. Turn them often. It takes about five minutes. Arrange them on the toast, add a little salt and a very little butter, serve very hot.

BROILED CHICKEN

The chicken must be young, split down the back. Lay on the gridiron and broil evenly, turning frequently. Serve on a piece of buttered toast, salt and slightly butter the chicken. A little parsley garnishes the dish prettily.

All birds to be broiled should be split down the back and broiled evenly, laid on thin toast and served hot.

BEEF STEAK

Steak must be cut 3/4 inch thick, and evenly broiled, rare, unless particularly requested to do otherwise. Be careful not to smoke it; the grease dropping into the fire may make trouble in this way.

OATMEAL GRUEL

Take two large iron tablespoonfuls of oatmeal freshly cooked for breakfast, add one cup of boiling water, slowly stirring all the time, then add an equal quantity of milk. Let all boil for ten minutes, and strain through a fine wire sieve. If you have no cooked oatmeal put 1/2 cup raw oatmeal in a double boiler with two cups of boiling water and cook for two hours, then proceed as above. It makes the gruel richer to add all milk, or 1-1/2 cups of milk and 1 cup of cream. Be sure not to forget the salt. Never put any sugar in unless requested to do it by the patient.

KOUMYSS

Dissolve a third of a cake of compressed yeast (Fleischmann's) in a little warm water (not hot). Take a quart of milk fresh from the cow, or warmed to blood heat, add to it a tablespoonful of sugar, and the dissolved yeast. Put the mixture in beer bottles with patent stoppers, fill to the neck, cork, and let them stand for twelve hours where the temperature is about 68 degrees or 70 degrees, then put the bottles on ice, upside down.

MILK PUNCH

One glass of milk, 1 or 2 tablespoonfuls of brandy, 2 teaspoons of sugar.

Shake well or beat with an eggbeater. Give cold. Have patient take slowly.

EGG-NOG

One egg, half glass of milk, 2 teaspoons of sugar, 2 teaspoons of sherry or brandy, ice. Beat the yolk of egg in a glass, add the sugar and beat, then a little milk, continue beating, then four or five pieces of ice about as big as a hickory nut; add brandy— regulate to the taste of your patient—add rest of milk; beat whites of eggs and add all but a teaspoonful with which garnish the top. It should make a glass brimming full. Have a spoon with which to eat it.

EGG LEMONADE

One egg, one-half a lemon, 2 teaspoonfuls of sugar, beat the white and yolk separately as for egg-nog; add the sugar to the yolk, then the lemon juice, then the ice, lastly the white beaten to a stiff froth.

WINE WHEY

One pint of boiling milk, one-half pint sherry; add sherry to the milk while scalding hot; stir a moment until the curd gathers; strain through a fine muslin, sweeten. To be taken cold. This takes a little practice to gather the curd as it should be done.

POACHED EGGS

The best way of cooking for an invalid. Slip the egg, previously broken into a saucer (the fresher the egg the better), carefully into salted water which is boiling in a frying pan, then immediately set the pan at the side of the stove so that the water does not boil, keep it there for about five minutes. Let the water be about two inches deep in the iron frying pan. Each egg must be broken separately and slipped carefully into the water. When cooked so that the white is firm but jelly like, no part being raw or hard, take it out with a skimmer and slip it on a piece of thin buttered toast, sprinkle a little salt and pepper on top, serve immediately. Garnish with parsley.

SCRAMBLED EGGS

Beat two eggs until thoroughly mixed, add two tablespoonfuls of milk, salt and pepper. Pour into a very hot frying pan, buttered, and stir constantly for about two minutes. Pour over buttered toast.

SHIRRED EGGS

Heat the shirring cup very hot. Put in a piece of butter as big as a large pea. Shake it about and break in the egg. Let it remain on the stove a few moments and serve in the shirring cup. Sprinkle salt and pepper on it.

OMELETTE

Beat very stiff two eggs, whites and yolks separately, add two tablespoonfuls of milk and a little salt. Pour carefully into a small frying pan, *hot* and buttered. As soon as the egg is *set*, slip a knife under one side and fold one side over the other. Slip on a piece of toast and serve at once. A little finely minced ham or parsley flavors it very well.

RENNET

One pint of milk slightly warmed and sweetened and flavored, add one large teaspoon of liquid rennet. Stir for a moment and set it in a refrigerator. To be eaten with sugar and cream.

BOILED CUSTARD

One pint of milk and 2 eggs. Beat the eggs, add the milk heated almost to the boiling point. Stir in 2 tablespoonfuls of sugar. Return to the double boiler, and cook for about 3 minutes, stirring gently all the time. When done it will be about as thick as cream. Be careful not to let it cook too much as it will "separate" and be spoiled.

BAKED CUSTARD

Same ingredients and proportions as for boiled custard, only let milk be cold. Pour into custard cups. Stand these in a dripping pan half full of warm water and bake in a pretty hot oven. Watch carefully, bake 15 minutes.

THIN BREAD AND BUTTER

Have a loaf of good home-made bread, yesterday's baking, cut off the crust, then butter the loaf and cut the slice in this way, buttering first and cutting afterwards. The slice can be made *very* thin and dainty, and the thinner it is, the better. A patient will sometimes relish this when tired of all kinds of toast or crackers.

VI
THE NURSE AS RELATING TO HER OWN TRAINING SCHOOL AND TO HER FELLOW NURSES

Always be loyal to your own school and hospital. It may not have been in every respect perfect; but it is not necessary to tell strangers of its imperfections: probably those in authority are just as sensible of its short-comings as you are, and perhaps they work harder than you do to right its wrong; in any case it does no good to tell others of the things you disapproved. It may indeed be that your criticism is one-sided and unfair, that the very rules you hated and found hard to keep are the wisest ones, and, if you let strangers see that you disapprove of these wise regulations, the opinion they will form of your intelligence will certainly not be flattering to you.

When you meet other nurses in your work, as you are sure to do, and when you compare your school with the one the other nurse came from, try to realize that the other school is neither wholly above nor wholly below your own; each has probably its own merits and its own drawbacks. You should not tell the other nurse any of your own school's shortcomings, any sooner than you would tell them to any other stranger; be loyal everywhere to the place where you were fitted for your work.

Never tell revolting hospital stories to your patients. Some people have the most morbid wish to hear dreadful details. I remember a patient of mine, years ago, asking me in all good faith to tell her the most horrible thing I had ever seen in all my hospital experience. I asked her why she wished to hear such things, and after some reflection she acknowledged that it was a foolish, morbid curiosity. It is best to keep the dreadful side entirely out of sight; there are plenty of bright, interesting, pleasant things always occurring; tell of these. Tell of the cunning little babies in the lying-in ward, the absurd little black ones, the fat little German and Swede babies. Tell of the surly drunken men that come, and how a week of cleanliness in bed, with a broken leg, or it may be a cracked skull, will change them into quiet, polite, pleasant patients; and how, later, they will take their turn at washing dishes, with a docility that would make their wives stupid with amazement. All such matters (and the more you try to think of them, the more you will be able to recall) will amuse and really edify your patient, many of whom think of a hospital only as a place of terror.

Never gossip about your sister nurses; of the stupidity of one, the untidiness of another, or the overbearing nature of the third. It can do no good, and it lowers you in the estimation of every one who hears you talk.

As for your duties to each other, I would have you always observe the same punctilious etiquette outside that you do in the hospital. When you are called to assist another nurse, remember that *she* is the head nurse; the case is hers. She gives directions, and you follow them; be sure you do it faithfully. If you have some one to assist *you*, be sure you arrange for her rest and exercise, and that you leave intelligently written orders when you go for your own rest.

Some very awkward complications may arise where there are two nurses, and the worst, I think, is for the patient and family to like the second nurse better than the first one, and to criticise her and find fault with her to the other nurse. This is hard all around. The second nurse expects the first one to be preferred, and usually dislikes to go to such a case, for that very reason; but if any of you find that under such circumstances you are preferred, never allow the people to retail to you the faults of the other nurse, and never gossip about her. She may not suit them, but she is probably doing the best she can, and such idle talk can do no good. If they *will* talk, make all the excuses for her you can, and never let her suspect from any action of yours, that you are preferred above her. If, on the other hand, you are the first nurse and some second one is called in, and preferred before you, study her well. See how it is that she wins the patient's confidence, when you did not. Try to find out, in a quiet way, wherein lies her charm. If it is quietness, exactness, cheerfulness, or ready tact—it must be something—and if you are clever you must see how it happens that she is preferred. It will be a good lesson for you. Perhaps you will never have such another chance for learning what you have found out by experience you lack. So do not waste your time by allowing yourself to feel jealous, but use it as a time of study, and you may reap a rich reward by winning your next patient's confidence.

VII
WHY DO NURSES COMPLAIN?

It seems to some of us, judging from the prevailing tone of nurses' conversations, that this is a veritable age of discontent. We hear that a nurse's life is confining; that it is wearing on the nerves; it keeps one from enjoying society; it is not sufficiently remunerative, etc., etc. We all know, without going into further particulars, what a nurse could complain about, and though each one's tale of woe may be perfectly true, it seems to me we are not wise, as nurses, to allow the trials of our professional life to occupy such a prominent position in our thoughts.

Let us glance at some of the other professions, and see how the members of each regard their chosen work. What is the prevailing theme of the religious newspapers? Is it complaints from the ministers that they are not appreciated, or that their life wears on their nerves? Not that surely, but we read of more and more work to be done; more and more need of the gospel to be preached and lived, that all may be attracted to it. What do we read in the medical journals? Not how often Dr. Jones or Dr. Smith has been called up at night, or how often they have been dismissed or maligned by ungrateful patients; neither do they talk of such things. Do they complain that they are kept from the presence of "Society?" Not so, and why? Their enthusiasm is such that these matters are accepted as part of the inevitable, and the higher, nobler aim is so real that the lower and meaner consideration of personal comfort sinks into insignificance. What is the soldier's favorite tale? Not that all through the war he had to drink his coffee without cream, that he did not have sheets on his bed, and that he ate from a tin plate. Would he ever speak of such things, except to show that a man can for a noble aim accept inconvenience, and laugh over it? Yet the soldier has probably been used to these comforts and many more all of his life in his home; but viewed in the light of his enthusiasm for the country he is striving to save, and seen by the side of her peril, such inconveniences sink into their merited nothingness.

Now the profession we have entered is, we are told, a noble one. We have been ranked shoulder to shoulder with the doctors, we have been compared to soldiers, we have been assured that our opportunities for doing good to souls are second only to those of the ministers. What more do we want? We want this, and we want it very much. We want the courage to accept our trials which must come if we are to have any glory. It is all very fine to be called a ministering angel, but it is pleasanter to minister to those who are appreciative. We *can* be heroic, in an emergency, but if we are not properly thanked, we do like to growl a little. It is gratifying to our vanity to be ranked with our masculine associates, but when it comes to the hard, thankless tasks which they accept without a murmur, then we proceed to show that we know what is what, and that our refined tastes cannot be so inconsiderately treated.

The trouble with these fretful nurses is that they *are* nurses. If they are not satisfied with the profession they have chosen, why do they not make a change and enter some other? Do they not know when they enter the work that it is hard, do they not hear on every side that it is exacting and confining? They knew it perfectly well before they began, why then do they complain? Why not say candidly, "I cannot have such enthusiasm for my fellow-men that I can forget myself," and then do something that is easier?

The Superintendent of the training school shows each new aspirant for the nursing profession that the life is not an easy one, that patience is one of the most necessary characteristics for the nurse. She tells her of the trials, the irritations, the unreason, the tiresomeness of sick people, and still women will come to the school, and forgetting the warnings, they will complain when some exasperating incident occurs. If a nurse, from overwork and the consequent weakening of her nervous energy, has lost her patience, she will be a wise woman if she drops out of nursing work for a year or more; this will probably help her, complaining never will.

Do you feel that your patient is cross or unreasonable? That is most likely, and is to be expected in nine cases out of every ten. Put yourself in your patient's place for a little while; try to realize what it is to have a pain, constant and sickening; to have it every minute of the twenty-four hours; try to imagine the fatigue of a respiration of forty; the ache and restlessness of a fever of 103 degrees; the agony of longing to change a position when it cannot be done; the despair of a hope for recovery growing daily less, or the realization of absolute weakness that comes with early convalescence; try to imagine yourself bearing some of these ills with nerves and brain weakened by disease, and you will not wonder that your patient is irritable, that he thinks the minutes of your absence are "hours," that the unevenness of the bed is "hard lumps," that the food is "slops," and the medicine "no good." Remember that he is a prisoner, and he has a cruel jailer; his bed is his prison, his disease is his jailer, and he suffers whatever torments his jailer chooses to inflict. Now prisoners are not, as a rule, a happy class of men; so bear with your prisoner and help him. Complaining about his shortcomings will never make them any the less. He is sick. Oh! the pathos of that short sentence, "He is sick;" that says all. You are well, or you ought to be; therefore bear with him.

You have chosen a hard profession, but we are told it is the noblest one a woman can follow. Why is it noble? Exactly because it is hard, and the hardness consists in your forgetting yourself and giving your strength to others. There are many hard lives that are not in the least noble, but there is no noble life that is not hard. A coal miner has, I suppose, a hard life, yet no one calls it a noble one; why? Because he works solely for his wages, and he complains and "strikes" when his wages and his hours do not suit him; but a doctor going from house to house, and in spite of all discouragements carrying cheer and hope; a city missionary going to the degraded, the ignorant, and by his own efforts helping his fellow-men to a better life, to a knowledge of God—these are noble lives. You can see I am sure the difference, and you will not gainsay me when I assure you that the doctor and the missionary, though they may not be satisfied with themselves, or with their manner of working, are happy men, happy because they live outside of themselves. The coal miner who is not content with his wages is miserable, because he himself and his needs loom up before him so large that every thing else is shut out. It is because you take a hard task and do it well, that so much praise is given to nurses. If you undertake a difficult task and fret over it all the time you are doing it, if you propose to benefit your fellow creatures and grumble because you have not comforts, or appreciation, or gratitude, where does the nobility go? Where is the heroism? If the task is easy, agreeable, delightful, the idea of heroism, of nobility, of all high aspiration dies directly. Did any one ever do a grand work and have an easy time while doing it? Did Florence Nightingale have all the comforts of life when she did her great work? Was it not by her indomitable perseverance, her great patience, and her enthusiasm for others that she won such an honored place for herself? You know almost before I say it, that there can be no loftiness of purpose, no enthusiasm, if there are not difficulties to be conquered, and you all know that complaining about sick people will never alter their characteristics, and that complaining about the nervousness of the relatives will never make less unreasoning, when they are fearful that a loved one is going to die.

Do we want gratitude and appreciation? We get it very often, and very often we do not; and when this last is the case, we may reflect that we are in very good company. How did the French reward Joan of Arc? The warmth of their gratitude led her to the stake. Galileo, as reward for his discovery, was put into prison and loaded with chains, as were also Christopher

Columbus and Sir Walter Raleigh, a notable company these, and every one suffered from the ingratitude of their fellow-men. Many more examples you must call to mind, of ingratitude more base than any thing we shall ever be called upon to bear.

The profession of nursing is still one of the most recent that women have engaged in. The world had until the past few decades been so used to being nursed by the old-fashioned nurse, who was a servant, and who never expected any treatment but that of a servant, that it has taken some years to always remember that we are not servants, in the usual acceptation of the term; but no one will be convinced of the fact that we are ladies by our *telling* them so. If you are a lady, with a lady's refinement, every one in the house will know it, will feel it, and you will never mention the subject; they must feel it, then there will be no arguing on the subject. It must be demonstrated by your deftness, your quietness, your cheerfulness, your education, your intelligence, your quick appreciation of other good qualities. We must all of us show the world that it is being nursed by its compeers, that a lady can do even the most revolting service in a way that robs it of its difficulties; and when the hard part of the illness is over, when your patient is ready and anxious to be entertained, you can show that you are not a machine for carrying out the doctor's orders; that you are capable of something more than the ability to take temperature, pulse, and respiration.

We must remember that even yet we are, in a way, pioneers of one part of that great woman movement in the world. It is not enough to educate one family up to the realization that we are its equals; the next house we go to, the same work may have to be done over again; but each time it is done, and done well, the whole profession has been benefited, which is an aim worth striving for.

VIII
THE NURSE AS A TEACHER

It does not occur to every nurse, when she graduates, that she has been preparing herself, during all these strenuous years of study and hospital work, for the life of a teacher. She fondly imagines that she is a nurse, and only that; but after she has been doing private duty for a year or more, she realizes that she is generally a teacher as well as a nurse, and that often she is a missionary also.

Perhaps no private duty nurse needs to be told what subject she must teach; the patient or the patient's friends never let her rest until she has told the "why" of every thing she does, or does not. There are, however, some important subjects that the nurse- teacher should try to make very clear to every patient.

We will begin with the baby, as the babies are with us always, and if doctors and nurses, science and sanitation have their way, there will some time be no call but that of the baby, for nurse or doctor either. The ignorance of the young mother is proverbial; her wish to know about her baby and its care is pathetically earnest. The new life is so precious, she would take such good care of it, if she only knew how. Here is a pupil eager for knowledge, ready to do all that can be intelligently taught to her. The nurse should have very clearly in her mind all the mysteries of digestion, all the reasons for regularity in feeding, the necessity for fresh air, for long and uninterrupted slumber, for loose clothing, for regular bathing. She should be able to give the mother the rules for her own living that she may be able to provide the best milk for the baby, or, if the little one has to be artificially fed, the methods of preparing the particular food chosen should be explained, and the indications of indigestion pointed out. All this is real teaching, real missionary work, and if well done will help the mother immensely and probably save the baby many attacks of colic or worse. Washing the baby is usually regarded by the young mother as a terrible ordeal. No nurse should leave her young-mother patient until she is fully able to perform this task. Let the mother watch, a few mornings, while the nurse does all the work, then let her undress the baby, when the nurse can take him and finish the operation. Day by day let her do a little more, as her strength and ambition permit, until at the end of a week she is fairly used to handling the child and can, perhaps, keep him until the last finishing touches are put on. The nurse should always be near, to help, to advise, to take the child should the mother become exhausted. Finally, she should go into another room, and, leaving all things ready, allow the mother to perform the duty by herself, letting her know that at any time she will be relieved if necessary. In this way the mother becomes accustomed to the child, and the bath is always a pleasure to her. How many times have we heard pathetic stories of a young mother trying for the first time to wash the baby?—the tears of despair, the nervous blunders, the exhaustion when the performance was brought to a hasty close. All such stories mean that the nurse in charge was not a teacher and that her work when she left the case was not completed.

Suppose that this baby is the third or fourth, the mother knows what to do for the new little one, but how about the others? She is still anxious to do what is right, or perhaps she is not anxious, and her attitude toward the children is not what it should be. Perhaps she does not realize that she will be called to account for these souls intrusted to her care, that these bodies will do their part in life, well or ill, as she treats them wisely or foolishly. Here is true missionary work. A thoughtful, intelligent, judicious nurse can show a mother that an adenoid may be responsible for Johnny's inattention, as it causes dullness of hearing, how Mary's fretfulness is caused by too little sleep or by insufficient ventilation of her room at night. She can explain how irregular eating causes the children to be cross and irritable. She can show why the first teeth should be removed when the second begin to push towards the gum. She can teach the mother that the headaches so often met with, in children who go to school, are due, perhaps, to eye strain, and can not be corrected with pills, and should never be soothed with headache powders. She can show the evils of the gallons of soda water too many young women swallow, of the injudiciousness of allowing young girls to congregate in drug stores. These last two evils, "soda water and the drug store habit," the mother may know nothing about. She is busy at home with the "little ones," and the fourteen- or sixteen- year-old girl only too often is allowed to wander off "down town" with other young girls, and what she does there would astonish many a mother.

Every nurse should know how to teach her patient to guard herself and her children from tuberculosis. She should be able to show what the early symptoms are, what is then necessary to do, what care should be taken of the sputum, of the patient's food, of his eating and drinking vessels, his bed and bedding. She should know how to teach a tuberculosis patient to care for himself, how he can avoid giving his disease to others, if he stays at home; and where he will find proper hospital or sanatorium accommodations if he goes away.

Most mothers are very thankful for practical hints from one who is supposed to know, and who, during a four to six weeks' stay, makes herself one of the family, and offers advice in the *right way* and *at the right time.*

The great sex question is almost sure to be discussed at such a time. The advent of a new baby is such a wonderful thing that nearly always the other little ones want to know (very naturally) where it came from. Little folks are brimful of curiosity. It is Nature's way, I suppose, of teaching them. Every new thing fills them with admiration, with joy, and they must know all about it. "Oh, mamma, what a lovely new pony! Where did you get it?" "Is it really mine?" "Oh, papa, what a dandy, new sled! Where did you get it? Can't I use it right now?" "Oh, have we got a new baby? A real baby? Is it ours? Where did it come from?" "Can't I hold it?"

All are familiar with these expressions of wonder, of delight, of joy of possession, but how to satisfy the eager mind aright is a problem requiring our most careful thought. Books, papers, and magazines tell us what to say and how to say it. All this should be talked over, and, if the mother does not know, the nurse should know what books to tell her to read.

The medical world to-day is much concerned over the question of prostitution and its effect upon the coming race, through the transmission of syphilitic taint to an innocent wife, who is thereafter barren, or who bears syphilitic children. The folly of the double standard, purity insisted on for the wife, unchasity condoned in the husband; all these subjects are sure to be brought up, and the nurse who goes prepared on these and kindred topics can do an immense amount of good to the women she nurses.

She can show how useful the knowledge of chastity is to a boy-the strength that comes from self-control, the weakness that follows self-indulgence, the danger to himself and to those he really loves when he contaminates himself with prostitutes. A young man once said to a friend of mine, "Oh! if my mother had only warned me of the suffering I would cause myself and others, I never would have polluted my body and shamed my soul." The nurse should know how to instruct the mother as to the signs of self-abuse in her little boys, so that she may know what causes the nervous movements, the pallor, the fitful appetite, the dark circles under the eyes, the listlessness, the fondness for being alone—any one of which should call for extreme watchfulness. All these things a nurse should be sure to know, so that, as far as in her lies, she should be one more earnest woman striving to make the world better for her having lived and worked in it. A wise man has given this quaint description of a perfectly educated man: "When a man knows what he knows, when he knows what he does not know, when he knows where to go for what he should know, I call that a perfectly educated man." So with the nurse. When she finds a social problem with which she is not familiar, let her turn to this list of books, magazine articles, and pamphlets upon the subject: Chapman, Rose R., The Moral Problems of Children; Dock, Lavinia L., Hygiene and Morality; Hall, Winfield Scott, Reproduction and Sexual Hygiene; Henderson, Charles W., Education with Reference to Sex; Lyttelton, E., Training of the Young in the Laws of Sex; Morley, Margaret W., The Renewal of Life; Morrow, Dr. P. A., Social Diseases and Marriage; Saleeby, Caleb W., Parenthood and Race Culture; Wilson, Dr. Robert N., The American Boy and the Social Evil, The Nobility of Boyhood, 50 cents (contained in "The American Boy and the Social Evil"); Hall, Stanley, Educational Problems, Chapter on the Pedagogy of Sex, Adolescence, Youth; Northcoate, H., Christianity and Sex Problems; Janney, Dr. Edward O., The White Slave Traffic in America; Report of the 3 8th Conference of Charities and Corrections, in Boston, June, 1911, Sex-Hygiene Section; Kauffman, Reginald Wright, The House of Bondage; Summary of the Chicago Vice Commission, in the May number of *Vigilance*; Education with Reference to Sex in the August number of *Vigilance* (published monthly at 156 Fifth Ave., New York City, at five cents per copy); The Cause of Decency, Theodore Roosevelt, *Outlook*, July 15, 1911; articles on The Causes of Prostitution in *Collier's Weekly*, from time to time, since April 1, by Reginald Wright Kauffman; articles on the Necessity for Teaching Sex Hygiene, in *Good Housekeeping*, beginning with the September number; Dr. Dale's articles on Moral Prophylaxis, in the JOURNAL OF NURSING since the July number; Instructing Children in the Origin of Life, Elisabeth Robinson Scovil, in October JOURNAL OF NURSING; Leaflets and pamphlets published by American Motherhood, 188 Main Street, Cooperstown, New York; Publications of the American Association of Sanitary and Moral Prophylaxis, New York City, JOURNAL OF NURSING, February, 1912.

One last word and I have finished. Be careful, oh so careful, that your instructions are acceptable, that your pupil is anxious to be taught. Most mothers are anxious on these subjects; if one is encountered who does not care, first try to make her care (and this is a task, indeed), and then teach her what to do and how to do it.

IX
CONVALESCENCE

One frequently hears the private duty nurse deplore the necessity of her remaining with a patient during convalescence. "I wish," such a one would say, "that I never need stay with a patient after the temperature has been normal for ten days," or, "I do not mind the first two weeks of an obstetric case, then there is something to do, but after that I am ready to leave," or again, "When my patient is ready to go out driving, I always wish she would drive me home; half-sick people are not to my taste." I have often wondered if this feeling is not caused by the atmosphere of the hospital which has, during training, been the nurse's home,—the hospital, where the patient leaves at the earliest possible moment of recovery, to make room for someone else. The pupil nurse gets used to the excitement of critical illness, used to the hard work of constant watching and fighting for the patients' lives, and that, and only that, it seems to her, is nursing. So when she goes to her private cases, and her patient has a long period of convalescence, she feels out of place, she does not seem to be doing what she was trained to do, and she frets over it, until some happy day when the doctor releases her, and she is at liberty to go once more to some one who is at death's door.

Nurses seem to feel that caring for a convalescent is not "nursing," but there they are mistaken. After a serious illness it takes a long time to restore the patient to perfect health, some function may need the close watching which only trained eyes can give, and it is not beneath the dignity of the nurse to remain, and keep watch until every part is once more in perfect working order. Many nurses feel that it is not nursing to amuse a patient, but it is nursing to help him on to the healthy plane from which he has fallen, to play games with an invalid and to watch him, to read with him, and to watch, to walk or ride or travel with him, and to watch, always to watch, that the dreaded symptom does not appear, that the one part which still needs care gets it.

A surgeon does not spend all day, every day, with his gloves on, and his scalpel in his hand; he is not *always* operating, or even arranging for operations; he can find time to see patients, to sit and talk with them, to advise them, to cheer them, even to tell funny stories to them, but all the time he is watching them. A lawyer is not always pleading in the court room, a clergyman is not forever in the pulpit. The lawyer when talking to his client is just as truly a lawyer; the clergyman, when visiting his congregation, is just as truly a clergyman,—the sermon on Sunday is the climax, if I may so express it, of his week's work. The lawyer's speech to the jury is the point to which all his efforts tend after, perhaps, weeks of preparation. So the convalescence of a patient is the post climax of the nurse's undertaking. She begins with the climax, severe illness, operation, or obstetric case, whatever it may be, gradually the stress lessens, the whole atmosphere of the house becomes natural as the patient progresses toward recovery; but the process is not complete, and the nurse's work is not done until the doctor pronounces her trained care no longer necessary; then she may go, and feel that her work has been thoroughly done-no small comfort surely.

I wish I could show my young sister nurses how good *for them* this period of the patient's convalescence might be. The delightful rest of regular sleep, and regular meals comfortably eaten at a table instead of in solitude from a tray, the opportunity for regular exercise—these things come as a real luxury when one has been nursing a critically-ill patient, and anxiety has been with one, night and day. This is the period when the nurse's nerves, strained to their utmost, can regain their tone, where the responsibility borne by the doctor and shared by the nurse is not so great a weight, and the knowledge of one more victory over death, one more human life saved, gives a joyousness to the day that is good to experience.

The satisfaction of knowing that by your help the patient has come, perhaps, from the gates of death; the pleasure of noting day by day the return of healthful sensations, the gradual ever- growing desire to once more take his accustomed place in the life work that has been interrupted—all these are missed by the nurse who flies from convalescents.

May it not be that the change in occupation has something to do with this unwillingness to remain with a patient when he is convalescing? When a temperature has to be taken but once a day, or when the doctor only makes visits twice a week, when all the routine of the sick-room gives way to a more natural atmosphere, many nurses do not feel at ease, they do not read aloud pleasantly, they do not care for books, and, if the patient asks for this amusement, the reading is a torment to the nurse, and I imagine it does not afford much pleasure to the listener. A nurse once gave me a graphic description of her efforts to read "Romola" to a convalescent typhoid patient. The poor nurse knew nothing of Florence or of the Italian language, and her struggles over the foreign words in that book must have been funny enough. Her patient was not much edified—of that I am certain. If a nurse does not read aloud understandingly, she should make every effort to learn.

She thereby increases her usefulness, and makes herself more acceptable to her patients. She adds to her own value. She is worth more. No nurse can tell when this method of passing the weary hours will be required of her, as it is almost certain that a patient of intelligence will ask for some mental refreshment.

Another pleasant way to pass the long hours of convalescence, is by playing games with your patient. I am sure no training school for nurses has added the study of cribbage, pinochle, bezique, chess, checkers, backgammon, or dominos to its curriculum. All these are two-handed games, the playing of which will help the convalescent to forget himself and his past illness and present weakness. The nurse, if she knows only one game that is unfamiliar to the patient, gives him new thoughts while she teaches him, and it is quite astonishing how much pleasure such simple things can give both to teacher and pupil. I would suggest that nurses in their club houses or homes could profitably fill some vacant evenings practising these two-handed games. I am sure they would never regret the time so spent.

If the convalescent is a woman, the means of amusing her are more varied and more congenial perhaps. In addition to reading aloud and playing games, there is the vast realm of "fancy work," where most women feel at home. It is a pity, so few women nowadays know anything about knitting, crochetting or tatting,—many do not even know which is which. A lady asked me very innocently, not long ago, how I could tell the difference between knitting and crochetting! Since Irish crochet has returned to favor, however, many have once more taken up their crochet needles. The nurse who can deftly turn her hand to these dainty arts, and can teach them to her patients, or any of the patient's family, has the means of making herself a very acceptable companion, apart from her nursing skill. Embroidery is very fascinating, and appeals to every woman. A dainty little garment for your patient, embroidered while you watch her return to health, will be long treasured by her. For a nurse, what art, what accomplishment can she have that will not help some poor invalid, that will not shorten the weary hours for some sick body, or bring consolation to a weary soul? A perfect nurse is one who brings comfort to her patient. It is because trained nurses bring more comfort that they have replaced the old style nurse; the more comfort the nurse brings, the more successful she is. The ability to talk well, when talk is needed, to read well, to amuse understandingly, to wisely meet each need of the invalid as it presents itself, this is to be the ideal nurse.

X
HOW SHALL A NURSE OCCUPY HER DAYS OF WAITING?

To many nurses the time between cases is dreaded as a period when money is being spent for necessary maintenance, and none is coming in; a nervous time, as the ring of the telephone which may mean a call is wished for or dreaded, perhaps both; an anxious time, as no one knows how long she may have to wait; a dreary time, as the days drag on and still no call comes. It *is* a trying time, but much can be done in these days of waiting that is delightful in the doing, and that will prove a source of pleasure to all future patients, and no little profit to the nurse also.

Let me preface my few hints by saying that all patients and patients' friends expect the nurse to know all about the diseases and their cures, the care and management of the sick,—that is common, ordinary nurses' business,—but there too many nurses stop; they often can go no further; and when one comes to a family and adds to this a broad culture, and an intelligent interest in the topics of the day, the respect and admiration of the patient and family are unbounded, and their surprise genuine.

I would like, if possible, to impress upon the nurse graduate that really there is much to learn after she has left the training school. All the technic of hospital and operating room is fresh in mind, but there is so much that lies necessarily outside the walls of a hospital, and this knowledge that comes with experience is a great part of what makes a successful nurse.

I will not touch here upon what every nurse knows so well, relating to the "preparedness" of clothes, satchel, and instruments. We take it for granted that all this is ready. The case before has been a hard one, we will imagine, and several days have been given to the luxury of whole nights in bed, and whole days of resting; this is all done, and the next case is awaited.

The best thing to do first is for the nurse to examine a little her mental equipment, see what she has stored away in her mind that can help the next patient, or that can assist in fighting the battle of hygienic cleanliness versus disease-bearing dirt. Let her consider whether she reads aloud acceptably, understandingly. Has she a good list of books which most women would enjoy? Does she know what books to suggest for the children? Can she tell what would interest the boys, or what a man would like to listen to? Does she know humorous books, interesting histories, or biographies? Here, then, is occupation for many idle days.

To go to a public library is always a pleasure, to make friends with the librarian is an added pleasure, as is also the making one's self familiar with some good books that can always be procured, and that will give pleasure and profit to patient after patient. This search for good literature will give happiness in the quest, and happiness in the reading. Librarians are usually glad to direct one to the books needed, and many delightful hours may be spent in the library, and all the while the comfortable feeling experienced that the pleasure felt will be transferred later to future patients.

The subject of hygiene is taught in most training schools, and indeed in many day schools as well; but this is a branch of knowledge that is growing so rapidly that, unless the very latest discoveries are learned, the nurse may find herself of use merely when the infection has done its work.

I wonder how many nurses have made use of the bulletins issued by the U. S. Department of Agriculture in Washington. These are called Farmers' Bulletins, but many of them are of use to all mankind, be they farmers or not. They are free to any who ask for them, and up to the present time about five hundred have been issued. They are upon all sorts of subjects—Flies, Malaria, The Destruction of Rats, Care of Food in the House, Fruit as a Food, Cereal Breakfast Foods, etc., etc., subjects *ad infinitum*. Here, then, is a mine of information open to anyone who asks; all one has to do is to write to the Secretary of Agriculture and ask to have sent a list of the Farmers' Bulletins published by his department, and from the list any bulletins may be selected, and they will be sent. Ask for what is needed; it is all meant for the education of the public. The information is absolutely reliable, and represents the best thought of the country—expert advice by the foremost scientists.

I have often thought that a nurse who made the nursing of children a specialty, or even those who nursed children occasionally, would be much profited by a course in a Kindergarten Training School. The private duty nurse, however, having but a few days at her disposal, cannot do anything as extensive as that; but a very good substitute is at hand, in the kindergarten department of any of our public schools. It is most interesting to go to a public school, ask to see the Principal, and let the nurse explain her visit, and show her how helpful it would be to future little sick folks, if she might be allowed to study some of the kindergarten methods, and permission will readily be given. When the nurse reaches the room of the "littlest ones," let her sit down, and quietly watch what is done for them, and how they are managed. The kindergartner will be glad to tell where she finds the charming stories she relates; she will give models of the wonderful things her pupils cut out of paper, the canoes, the men to sit in them, the wigwams, the sleds, automobiles, swings, stoves, trees, apples, etc., etc., articles well-nigh innumerable, and all so simple and so deftly made. A small convalescent could be amused for weeks with the things one could learn in a few hours in one of our city kindergartens. I speak of the things I know, for I have tried it, and I never yet found a Principal who was not glad to have her kindergarten studied, nor a kindergartner who was not pleased to know that she could assist in the work of nursing sick children, even in this seemingly roundabout way.

In all of our large cities are fine art galleries, and in many there are fine loan collections on exhibition every summer. There are, besides pictures in these loan collections, many things; some curious, some beautiful, and all of them interesting. Some days spent in these galleries will bring much knowledge and beauty into one's life. Time must be taken for these visits; no one can appreciate the patience and skill of oriental handiwork in a hurry. If unacquainted with the exhibits, a catalogue should be purchased, and each one studied until one knows why it is there, and what is its beauty. I remember seeing, one day, in a collection, a cup of jade, with a very finely wrought handle; I thought it fine, but did not appreciate it until the Custodian told me that it took the artist twenty years to carve that one cup, jade is such a hard stone. This cup was so valuable that the Kensington Museum, in England, had paid an immense sum of money for it, as a nearly perfect specimen. This information was my reward for close study of an exhibit. In these exhibitions one could spend many vacant days with much pleasure and profit.

In whatever town a nurse lives she should familiarize herself with the philanthropic efforts of the place. In the largest cities it is not possible to know them all, but she should know about some of the settlement work, the day nurseries, the babies' hospitals, the rescue work, the homes for aged. Of course she will know about the hospitals and dispensaries, but what is done for the poor, the ignorant, the sinful, and the stranger—these she should learn. Many times she could do much to help these institutions, by relating, simply and truthfully, when occasion offers, what she has seen, of the great needs of such efforts, and the heroic work of those who go down and live amongst the needy and try to uplift them. Many a rich, idle patient might become interested and give money, if not time, to help in these good works; and my experience shows that they generally need all the help they can get. So the nurse should know about the anti-tuberculosis work, the night schools, the playgrounds on the roofs of the school-houses, all the philanthropic work of her town, and she cannot know about it unless she takes some of her vacant days, her days of waiting, and turns them into days of learning, and the expansion of both her mind and her heart.

Another pleasant way to spend some days of waiting is to study the trolley system of the town where you live. Learn how far it can go, to how many other towns. If a river is near, become familiar with its steamboats. Excursions on boat or trolley will be delightful, and will teach the best routes, the best terminal stations, and the best restaurants, and some day when a patient is well enough to take an excursion, some part of his own immediate neighborhood may be shown him which he has never seen before. Believe me, all this will be appreciated. Space fails me to tell of music to be heard, theatres to be enjoyed, and all to be used hereafter for the benefit of those to whom you will be called to minister. The information constantly gathered in the "days of waiting," rightly used, intelligently imparted to the patient or her friends, will make of the nurse such a broad-minded, sympathetic woman that everyone who employs her will appreciate the fact that she has a wide culture, and brings to her patient something besides mere technical skill.

XI
SOME HINTS FOR THE OBSTETRICAL NURSE

THE BABY'S WARDROBE

When a nurse goes to see a woman who wishes to engage her, some months hence, to care for her baby and herself, it is very nice to be able to give her, should she ask, a list of all the things she will need, both for her own comfort and the baby's.

The following is a good sensible wardrobe, and will be found ample, though many articles more or less fanciful will, most probably, be added by friends. The things enumerated below should last the baby until he is put into short clothes:

Slips, 10. Dresses, 8 to 10. Pinning blankets, 4. Flannel skirts, 4. White skirts, 5. Shirts, 4. Bands, plain flannel, 4. Bands, Jersey made, 4. Diapers first size, 17 inches square, 20. Diapers second size, 20 inches square, 30. Diapers third size, 26 inches square, 30. Knitted blankets, plain white, 2; if with any color, 4 to 6. Knitted sacques, 4 (two sizes). Little pillow (hair), 6 cases. Crib sheets, 6. Crib blankets, 2.

FOR BASKET

Two small gold safety pins. Large safety pins, I box. Small safety pins, i box. Powder box and puff. Coudreay's powder. Small box of equal parts borax and powdered sugar. Old damask towels. One cake old white castile soap, or Colgate's nursery soap. One bottle unscented vaseline. As many sachets as you can get. Some few yards of the narrowest ribbon, pink and blue. Two old handkerchiefs. One lap protector. Brush and comb. Absorbent cotton.

FOR THE MOTHER

All the old sheets in the house. Rubber sheet, double width. A square of rubber sheeting single width. An old comforter. [Footnote: When the Kelly pad is used for the delivery, the old comfortable, the blankets and the single width rubber sheet need not be provided.]Two or three old blankets. Fountain syringe. Paper basin. Towels ad libitum. Six or seven night dresses, three of them old. Undershirts, if worn in bed, 4 (large). Bandages,

6. Cheese cloth, 10 yards. Absorbent cotton, 2 lbs. A large flannel sacque, or a nightingale. Soft unbleached muslin, 2 or 3 yards. Colgate's fumigating wafers, I box. Bedpan, I.

Layettes can be purchased at any good department store, but many expectant mothers prefer to make all the clothes for the little one. These lists are for the benefit of these mothers.

These look, perhaps, like two very formidable lists, but a second glance will convince any one that all these articles are absolutely necessary, and none of them are expensive.

The slips should be made very plainly. The material may be as fine as can be bought, but beyond a few tucks about the yoke, and a little lace or fine embroidery about neck and sleeves, should be perfectly plain. The dresses, of course, are somewhat more elaborate, but the fashion now decrees that infant's clothing shall be perfectly plain, and a most sensible fashion it is. Pinning blankets are open all down the front, and are usually made in the shops with a broad band of stiff white muslin, which shows that the people who made them never tried to dress a baby. The band should be of flannel or coarse linen many times washed so that it may be soft, and the pins will go through many folds of it. Flannel skirts are usually made of two breadths of flannel, and are more or less embroidered. These are not left open, except just enough to make the dressing easy. Shirts are made so well in stores that few people care to knit them. They should always be high in the neck and long sleeved, and it is better to get two sizes, as, if the baby is small, it never can be comfortable in a large shirt that does not fit.

The four flannel bands should be 6 inches wide by 17 or 18 long, torn the length way of the flannel and left just as torn. Not hemmed or ornamented in any way. No hemming or stitching can be so fine that it will not mark the baby's flesh. Besides this, if you have these plain bands and find they are several inches too big, nothing is easier than tearing off a strip and making them fit. If the child has a very large, round abdomen, they can be made to fit over it nicely by taking two little tucks on the lower edge, about half an inch from the middle of the band, and letting the tucks run up about an inch or a little more, tapering it off gradually. When these are discarded and the Jersey made bands are put on, always put them on the baby feet first, as it is hard to get them over the shoulders.

The very best material for the first small diapers is old, soft table damask. The better the quality, the softer it will be; be sure they are exactly square. Nothing is more trying, in a small way, than to get a diaper that cannot be folded true. These should be made double and the edges turned in and sewed around. By the time the baby has outgrown them they will be fit only for the rag- bag, and may be thrown aside. The second size diaper, also the third should be many times washed to make them soft enough for use. These may be used at first folded eight times and put under the baby next the damask diaper, between that and the pinning blanket, and will often save the nurse the trouble of changing the baby's clothing, because it is wet through. In this way they will get more washings and be softer when you have to use them next the baby's skin.

Cotton flannel, with a good nap and not a very close web, is very good also and can be used instead of the damask where that cannot be procured. Put it on with the nap next the skin. It is an excellent absorbent.

The baby should have at least one little (rather flat) hair pillow, covered on one side with blue or pink silk, on the other with plain white over the ticking. The prettiest pillow cases I ever saw were made of broad hemmed pocket handkerchiefs. Two sewed neatly together round three edges, and on the fourth button holes for mother-of-pearl studs. The handkerchiefs may be fine or not, embroidered or plain, and may have lace sewed on the edge, but they can't help being pretty, and the embroidery will never be in the middle. I shall never forget my pity for one poor little mite I saw once, who, on waking from his sleep, was discovered to have the print of an embroidered S on his cheek. It had been worked in the centre of the little pillow case by some loving but ignorant hands. When the baby uses the pillow, let him sleep on the white side; at other times turn up the colored side and the pink or blue will show very prettily through the linen. If you let the child sleep on the colored side he may, most likely will, vomit some sour milk on it, sooner or later, and the beauty of your pillow will be gone.

If the regular little crib blankets are thought too expensive, a very good substitute may be made from white eiderdown cloth, which is warm, soft, and not at all costly.

The gold safety pins are intended for the final pinning of the dress in the front and in the back. Of course any little ornamental baby pin answers the purpose just as well, and, indeed, an ordinary safety pin will do should no other be at hand.

The little box of equal parts of borax and sugar should not be forgotten. Mix the two very thoroughly, and if any little white aphthous spots appear on baby's lips, tongue or cheeks, apply a little of this mixture several times a day, and they will probably all be gone by night. Put it on very carefully with the tip of your finger slightly moistened so that some of the powder will adhere. Examine the baby's mouth every day for these spots. They are likely to appear any time after ten days or two weeks, and are more often seen in weak children, or those who are fed by a bottle. If the spots appear on a child who is taking the breast, the nipples are very apt to be sore. Much care, therefore, must be exercised in this matter.

Sachets are a real luxury in the drawers of the baby's bureau. Atkinson's sachets are the best, though Colgate's violet is very delicate and pleasant. Put one or two amongst the little shirts, and some among the knitted blankets, but mostly have them in the dresses, and be sure when you take out a clean dress, or slip, to take the sachet and slide it into the neck of the slip that will be worn tomorrow. Nothing can be more attractive than a clean, sweetly smelling baby, and, *per contra,* nothing is more disgusting than a wet, sour, cold, crying baby. If he be wet and sour he will surely have cold feet and hands, and as surely will he cry. Poor little thing! It is his only way of expressing his opinion of the state of his toilette.

It is very pretty, when the baby is fresh and clean, and has on a fine slip with lace edging the sleeves, to tie around the wrist, outside of the sleeve, a piece of pink or blue ribbon. Make a nice little bow and let the lace fall over the fat little hands, like a frill. Be careful not to tie the ribbon too tight, and keep it clean. If it becomes soiled or wet, take it off directly.

A lap protector is made by covering a piece of rubber cloth about 14 inches square with several thicknesses of old blanket. To cover this have some slips like pillow cases, of linen or cotton, plain or fancy, as the lady may have time or money. Slip the "protector" in its case, and lay it on your own, or any one else's, lap who wishes to hold the baby, and it perfectly protects from all wetting.

TABLE FOR ESTIMATING THE PROBABLE DURATION OF PREGNANCY

Two hundred and eighty days, forty weeks, ten lunar months, or nine calendar months are here estimated as the usual duration of pregnancy (the actual computed average being 276-2/3 days). The exact day of conception (*not* the fertile coition), can never be accurately determined; the only date from which conception can be dated, and the probable confinement day predicted with some chance of certainty, is the first day of the last menstrual flow, adding to this one week (seven days) for the average duration of the flow (with a few days lee-way). We count nine calendar months forward, and have the approximate date of the expected confinement. The most ready method is to add seven days to the first day of the last menstrual flow, count back three months, and add one year, when we have the future date when, or about when, delivery may be expected.

An *exact* estimate is but guess work; errors of one or two weeks either way may be made by the most experienced, as in cases where conception occurred shortly before the next menstrual period, which did not then appear.

The present table is constructed on the above principle, the second column representing the day of quickening, nineteen weeks after the beginning of the last menstruation, with seven days added; and the third column still twenty weeks later. The date of quickening is still more variable than that of delivery, from one to four weeks.

Intermediate dates may be fixed by adding the necessary number of days to each column. Thus, for Jan. 11th, the second column should read 31st of May, and the third column, October 18th, and so on.

Beginning of last Quickening. Confinement. Menstruation.

Jan. 1st.........May 20th.........Oct. 8th.
Feb. 1st.........June 20th.........Nov. 8th.
March 1st.........July 18th.........Dec. 4th.
April 1st.........Aug. 18th.........Jan. 6th.
May 1st.........Sept. 17th.........Feb. 5th.
June 1st.........Oct. 8th.........March 8th.
July 1st.........Nov. 17th.........April 7th.
Aug. 1st.........Dec. 18th.........May 8th.
Sept. 1st.........Jan. 18th.........June 6th.
Oct. 1st.........Feb. 17th.........July 8th.
Nov. 1st.........March 20th.........Aug. 8th.
Dec. 1st.........April 19th.........Sept. 7th.

ARTICLES FOR THE MOTHER'S USE

Perhaps it is not necessary to say why it is better to use old sheets for the bed of a parturient woman, but I will repeat that old ones are to be preferred, and really new ones, that is, only once washed, never used. New towels are of course objectionable, as being too harsh. If the patient likes a rough towel, use a regular bath towel, if you can get it. Be careful, never to let loose and wet ends of the wash cloth drag along exposed parts of the body. It is a good plan to sew your wash cloth into a bag, and to slip your hand inside, and work with it put on like a mitten. A rubber or fibre sponge is to be preferred. Keep one for the face, neck, arms, and hands, and another for the feet and legs. The vulva is bathed best by means of a fountain syringe used as an irrigator, and a little sterilized gauze twisted around your dressing forceps. The gauze can be changed as often as necessary, and is much more satisfactory than anything else, especially if there has been a laceration.

The square of rubber sheeting, single width, is most useful. For the confinement the bed should be made by first spreading over the mattress the wide rubber sheet, over this put an old blanket, then the under sheet; upon the right side of the bed, where most likely the woman will lie, place the square of rubber, over that the old comfortable, four double, and hold all in place with a sheet folded like a hospital "draw-sheet." This must be firmly tucked in at the sides under the mattress. It will seldom be found necessary to change the under sheet, if the bed is made this way, and the rubber square is drawn carefully away, with the comfortable and draw sheet, when it is time to make the patient clean and dry after the birth. It is a good plan now to tear this square in two, and keep one piece directly under the clean draw sheet for the first few days. This saves much washing.

An old blanket and a small one will be found invaluable for all sorts of things—for example, to spread over the shoulders and chest when the bandage is being pinned; to warm and wrap up the feet and legs, if they show any signs of being cold; to cover one knee and part of the body when using the irrigator, which when there has been *any* laceration, is a delicate piece of business, as every nurse knows. Always fold up this invaluable and constant friend, and put it in some handy but inconspicuous place; it *is* a friend, and a good one; but it is not a beautiful object to look upon, and others not knowing its virtues would think you untidy if it was in a noticeable place. The fountain syringe is absolutely indispensable; and, though it may seem unnecessarily large, yet I think a four-quart bag better than any of the smaller sizes. To be sure, you never might need four quarts in the bag, but it is so much easier managed, so much less liable to spill over, if you have a large bag and put it only half or three-quarters full. Then, too, you get so much more force if you have more water in the bag, you need not use it all. A Davidson syringe is very nice for some things that a fountain syringe could not be used for. Oil enemas, for instance, also nutritive enemas. After an oil enema be sure to wash your syringe *thoroughly* with a strong solution of washing soda or ammonia, else you will find the rubber of the bulb and tubing becoming pasty, and your syringe will be utterly spoiled. The paper basin is very light and easily handled and much to be preferred to a large china affair, which may easily slide from warm, wet, slippery hands.

I often wonder that the women of our day, who are so sensible in many things, should have abandoned the fashion of short night gowns, which our grandmothers always provided for themselves at these times. I remember asking one lady, when talking over what she would need for her first baby, and for herself, at the time of its birth, if she had not something short and plain that she could wear. She looked very thoughtful for a moment and then said that she thought she did have *one* night-dress that did not have a ruffle or embroidery around the bottom. She could wear that. It certainly is not from motives of economy that our wealthy patients do not have these most sensible of garments. I think they know nothing about them, and they should have their virtues explained to them. A pocket could be added to this garment, I think, and it would be a real comfort to a woman. I know it would be to a nurse, who usually has to hunt up the ever missing pocket handkerchief a dozen times a day. Men always have pockets in their night-shirts, and they are not sick half as much as the women. I wonder why women do not imitate this most sensible custom. If your patient will not let you cut off any of her old night-dresses, you must use the long ones, of course, and change them as often as necessary.

Bandages should always be made of soft unbleached muslin; double is best, though I have used them of the single fold, and hemmed, but they are firmer if double. They should be wide enough to come down to the great trochanters, and up to a place two inches above the umbilicus; long enough to fit the woman before she became pregnant. She has likely some measure, or could get it from her dress-maker. Women vary so much, it is hard to give an exact measure in inches, but you might begin with a bandage fifty inches long, and if the ends are too long, cut them off, and turn in the edges of the cloth and overhand it neatly.

Obstetrical binders, or bandages are now seldom put on a parturient woman, but in case they are to be used, I give the best kind I know of. They are sometimes made to order, but I never knew one of these to fit, or wash well.

The method of their application is of course taught in the schools. The nurse should always know from the doctor, or the prospective patient, if binders are to be worn, and instructions given as to how to make them. Four or six will be enough.

Two or three yards of soft, unbleached muslin for breast-bandages should be provided in case they are needed. A six-tailed bandage is, I think, the best for this purpose. Tear down the first two "tails" to within three inches of the others, and these passing over the shoulders, and fastening to others, which are adjusted over the breasts, keep the whole bandage in place.

It is not necessary to speak of the napkins or pads; these are universally used, and readily bought, sterilized, and ready for use. All sterilization is so thoroughly taught in the schools, I have taken proficiency in this particular for granted.

There should always be a disinfectant or antiseptic of some sort on hand.

Carbolic I-30, Platt's chlorides, permanganate of potash, or something that will answer the purpose; bichloride of mercury, etc. You must find out from the physician which he prefers, and of what strength.

I must not forget to say that when you go to see you prospective patient, and she shows you the room she expects to occupy, it would be well to cast your eyes about for some rug, that you can, if necessary, turn wrong side out and spread at the side of the bed. Some doctors are very neat about their work, but some are— well, perhaps I better not say it; we must not criticise the doctors.

But sometimes it is best to have protection for the floor, it gives the nurse a comfortable feeling quite beyond description to know, that, no matter what may happen, the carpet will not be ruined.

XII
AS TO WASHING THE BABY

In the first place get together everything you will need for the bath and subsequent dressing. Have the clothes all laid in order over a chair-back before an open fireplace, or over a radiator, or if no better expedient suggest itself, fill bottles with hot water, or get a hot water bag and fill that, and lay it *over* the clothes arranged in the order you will need them, beginning the pile with the dress and having the band the last. Have *two* large, soft towels and keep them warm. If possible, have an apron made of rubber cloth to tie about your waist. At your side, on the floor, have a small blanket ready to lay over the rubber apron when needed. Put your baby basket where you can reach it, be sure that it contains all the things you will need—sponge, soap, powder, pins, vaseline, etc., and an extra diaper or two. Now get the tub (tin) and pour in the water until it is about four inches deep. Have the water no warmer than 100 degrees F. Bath thermometers are made that are quite cheap, and a great convenience; one should always be at hand, as no nurse should ever trust her feelings as to whether the water is hot enough or not. Always test any water to be used for the sick or the delicate with a thermometer. Another point a nurse should be most careful about, is to be careful that her hands are warm before she takes the baby, as her cold hands on his warm flesh will surely make him scream.

All being now ready, take the baby and sit down with him, spreading the blanket over your knees as you do so, and having the tub just in front of you on another chair. The sponge is best to use for the washing, but a piece of old table damask is very good. Wash the eyes very carefully first, then the face, and dry on the towel. Now hold the baby's head over the tub and give that a good washing with soap on your bare hand, and rinse it well with plenty of water, always holding the left hand under the head and neck. Bring him back on your lap and thoroughly dry his head, then wash and dry the ears carefully.

When you get this far you may undress the baby completely, being most careful yet not taking any unnecessary time. When he is quite ready for the tub, grasp him firmly with the right hand, letting the buttocks rest in the palm of the hand, the fingers being outspread, and the thumb coming up almost to the pubic bone. With the left hand hold the head and shoulders. Lower him *very* gently into the water. Any sudden movement is most injurious, as a baby must never cry when the band is off, if it can be avoided. He will often put out both hands as if trying to catch hold of something. If he seems frightened at the same time, and cries violently, let the buttocks rest on the bottom of the tub, and with the right hand hold both of his, and he will be comforted.

I think it well to wash the whole body with your bare hand, well soaped. Be careful to wash under the arms, in the bend of the elbows, the groins, and under the knees, rinse him with the wash cloth or sponge, and now lay one warm towel on your lap, and take up the baby just as you put him in, slowly, and without shock, and lay him in the warm towel. Lay the second one over him, and draw over all the blanket, wrapping him up warm and snug. Put your hand inside the blanket and dry him. This can be easily and quickly done without at all uncovering the child. Pass the hand with a slight squeezing movement over each arm and leg, and over the front of the body. When this is done, you must undo the blanket, and take the upper towel and dry most carefully all the creases, and powder everywhere, especially if he is very fat. Get down to the very bottom of every crease, and be sure it is dry and powdered. Lay over the navel a compress of absorbent cotton, unless the child is over four weeks old, and over this the band, which should be unhemmed, and wide enough to extend from the hip to the armpit. Lay the palm of your right hand firmly over band and pad and turn the child carefully, holding your right hand still under him, and with the left, clear away all damp towels, and then straighten out the band that is wrinkled under one side. Keep your knees close together. Now take away the right hand, and see that the baby's knees are on the right side of your knee, and the elbows well over the other side of your lap. Now you have the baby where he can kick, but he can't wriggle or spring off your lap. See that the back is dry, rub it a little with your hand, and powder. Look carefully in the deep dimple just at the coccyx and see if it is clean. Now pin the band snugly, but not too tight. Use the smallest safety pins, and never pin directly over the spine. Sometimes the abdomen is very large and it will be necessary to make two little tucks in the lower edge of the band in front to make it fit snugly.

While the baby is still on his stomach, lay in place the diaper, and next the shirt, which should be open in the front, and the pinning blanket. Lay all of these just as they should be, as regards the back, and turn him, being careful to hold all the clothes in place. If he is liable to chafe, or the movements of the bowels are in any way irritating, use vaseline about the buttocks. Now put the arms in the shirt sleeves and tie or button it up, and then pin the petticoat or pinning blanket. Lay an extra diaper folded many times under him, and fold the pinning blanket just in three, bring the hem up to the waist and pin in place.

The dress goes on feet first. Slip it on over the pinning blanket, and pass the right hand up under the buttocks, and with the left, pull the dress into place, put the little hands in the sleeves, and get it perfectly straight and smooth over the chest. Now pass the fore-finger of the left hand down inside of all the clothes, beginning at the neck, until you find the band (the first garment), take a small safety pin or any small ornamental pin, and pin thoroughly through everything. This last pin I consider most necessary, as it keeps the dress, shirt, band and all in place. Turn the baby over once more and put a similar pin in the back of the dress, being very careful to get at the band. While the baby is in this position put the blanket he wears during the day over him, and a final turn brings him around, and he is washed and dressed all but his mouth, which must be carefully washed with clean, warm water or borax and water. This should be also done many times each day, if the mouth is sore, and always a sharp watch kept for white patches on lips, cheeks and tongue. If the baby has hair to brush, it is well to brush it. It makes him look very cunning, but if he is tired or sleepy, do not trouble him. This washing and dressing should not occupy more than twenty minutes, I have done it in fifteen where the baby was very well behaved.

Be sure that the room is warm and that the windows and doors are kept closed. Do not allow admiring relatives to come and go, opening and shutting the doors as they do so. If they want to see the operation, let them come and stay. A baby should never be bathed in a tub until the stump of the cord is off and the navel well and strong. If there is any inclination to pouting of the navel, wash the child on your lap and do not take off the band until the rest of the baby is all washed, dried, and powdered. Then take off band and compress, and put on fresh ones as quickly as possible, turn the child and pin as before directed.

In taking the clothing off, it is not necessary to turn the child at all, the band being the only thing pinned in the back.

N. B.—This method of bathing is for a normally healthy child, from the time it is one week old, until it is six months or more.

Until the stump of the cord has sloughed off, a baby should never be put into the tub. If after the stump has sloughed there seems to be any protrusion, or indeed any ulcerated look about the naval, it is best to bathe the child on your lap. In all such cases undress the baby as previously directed, until you come to the band (flannel belly band). Wash, rinse, wipe and powder him, being careful to make every part absolutely clean and dry. If the band is soiled or wrinkled, or out of shape in any way, remove it and put on a fresh one—looking every day, after three days, to see if the stump has come off—and if it is still adherent, being most careful not to disturb it in any way. Apply the fresh band immediately. Turn the baby on its stomach, and when the back is exposed, wash and rub the back gently with your warm hand. If the band does not need changing, unpin it, rub the back, pin it up again, and proceed in dressing as before. When the cord is once fairly off, and the navel smooth and clean, you can put the baby into the tub, very gently, slowly, and cautiously, remembering that a sudden movement on your part may, in fact, always will make him scream, and screaming with no band or compress on is for a baby a very frequent cause of umbilical hernia. If the cord is small when the child is born, there will be less danger of hernia, but if it be a large one, then beware! It will not always be your fault if the baby's navel is not small and flat when you are leaving your case, but you will always be blamed for it, if it is not. Notice carefully every morning when you bathe the child if there is any umbilical protrusion, and report it without delay to your doctor, if there is any, no matter how slight. This is not, however, the place to treat of umbilical hernia, and we will go on with the washing, If the child's skin is very tender, chafing easily, wash with castile soap suds, rinse and dry carefully, after every time he urinates, as well as when you bathe him. Powder with talcum powder. Sometimes no powder will do it any good, then try vaseline. If that will not do, ask the doctor if you can try oxide of zinc ointment. Ordinarily, extreme care in washing, drying and powdering will be sufficient, but it must be done every time the diaper is changed. In this, as in other things, eternal vigilance is absolutely necessary.

When the baby is about two or three weeks old, it is a good plan to put some alcohol into the water in which he is bathed—two or three ounces to the amount of water used in bathing. Have a small bowl of cooler water, 70 degrees to 80 degrees, for the face, and after that is washed, add a tablespoonful of alcohol to that also, for the head. It helps to toughen the skin, and prevents the baby from taking cold so easily.

If the baby seems much frightened by being put into the tub, spread a bath towel or small thin blanket over it and have someone hold his hands, so that he will not clutch so wildly at everything, then lower him into the water, towel and all, and he will not notice it so much.

I know of no place where deftness of handling shows to such advantage as with a baby. He knows well enough if he is handled properly or not, and his fretful cry, or violent screams, will tell you without delay if he is not comfortable.

Once more, let me impress upon the minds of all who read this, the necessity of having everything used about the tub and subsequent dressing, warm. Anything cold will make the little one scream, and I think all nurses will agree with me, that there is no more nervous work than washing and dressing a baby who is crying (and once he begins, he is only too apt to keep it up during the entire time). This is especially true if a weak, ignorant mother is made nervous by the noise, or a doting grandmother hovers about, making remarks about "new fashioned ways," and wondering why this child should cry when his mother was always so good, as a baby, in her bath.

Now, as to the time of washing a baby. The morning is unquestionably the time, but if the baby be very young (less than two weeks) and has been wakeful during the night, I would let him have his nap, even if it did delay you and interfere with your plan of work. If he sleeps he is comfortable, and, unless for some more serious reason than the bath, he ought not to be disturbed. This, for babies in private practice. Hospital babies cannot be so tenderly cared for. When there are ten or eleven to be washed in one morning, choose, of course, the ones that are awake, as far as you can, but there will always be one or two sleepy, warm little ones about whom you will have some twinges of conscience as you begin to wash their faces, but the work presses so, it must be done.

A baby should not be bathed just after nursing, or when he is hungry. Yet, most little babies go to sleep at the breast, and very often do not waken until they are once more ready for eating. This seems like stating a difficult problem, and I know it is not always easy to select just the proper time, but the best way, I think, is this.

If the baby is nursing from the breast, tell the mother, after this nursing you wish to wash the child, and not to let him go off for sound sleep. She can prevent it, and keep him for the twenty minutes or half an hour it is necessary to wait after his meal, meantime you have time to get everything in readiness for the bath. It is a great mistake to attempt to bathe a baby when he is hungry. He will scream for his food from the beginning to the end of the performance, hesitating occasionally when something warm touches his mouth, and he eagerly seeks his meal, only to redouble his cries when not satisfied. Nothing is so persevering in its endeavors, as a hungry baby. Satisfy its appetite first and wait a reasonable length of time, wash him deftly and quickly, and he will be so sleepy by the time you are through, you can lay him in his bed and he will be asleep in a moment, when you can pick up all the soiled clothing and the general "mess" of the bathing operation, and leave the room once more tidy.

And just here, let me say a little about the washing of the baby's clothes. Of course the dresses or slips, skirts, and the diapers go to the laundress. Begin every morning on an entirely new, that is newly-washed, set of diapers. Gather up all that have been used the past twenty-four hours and have them washed. Perhaps they may not be ironed, but washed they should be, every twenty-four hours, even if you have to do it yourself, and I do not think a nurse should ever be called upon to do this. Still, I would rather do it than use a diaper over and over again.

But it is of the little shirts I particularly wish to speak. I think the nurse should wash these, also the socks when they need it, and the knitted shawls most babies wear. It takes very little time to do this, and if you know how, you will do it much better than any laundress. The best way to wash these things is in cool borax water, and if there is any one place the baby has vomited on, put a little dry powdered borax on (the place being wet), and rub it in. Then wash by plunging it in the water and squeezing it out. Do this again and again until the garment is clean. Rinse in clear cool water, and wring as dry as possible in a towel; then pull in shape and lay it on a clean towel to dry. It is a good plan to lay it on a folded towel over a half shut register and place a single fold of towel over. It will dry very soon. If you are washing a baby's knitted shawl, be very careful about the wringing. Lay a large towel (bath towel is the best) out flat, and, having squeezed the most of the water from the blanket, lay it carefully on the towel and roll both together, and wring very tightly. If this towel gets wet take a second. When you are satisfied that it is as dry as you can make it, lay it out on a folded sheet on the floor, in some room not much used, and pull and arrange it into its original shape and size.

Anything made of Germantown wool stretches terribly, but you can arrange it as it ought to be. It will look ruffly here and there and ridgy all over, but when it is dry it will shrink down all right. Only do not hang it up, and when it is dry you will be surprised to find it looks as good as new. If you are ever consulted beforehand as to what would be nice for the baby, use all your eloquence against *any* color being put into these knitted shawls. Germantown wool is the best to use, and plain knitting or brioche stitch is the best to wear and wash, and these things must be washed with the most careful handling. On the nicest baby they will become dirty, and the delicate blues and pinks become the dismalest wrecks when washed. Therefore, tell your patient not to put any color in these first plain little comfortable shawls. They should be a yard long by about three- quarters wide. Two or three will be all you will need, and do not use any of the fancy blankets sent in by friends. Lay these all away, with a sachet bag or two, in some convenient drawer, and never take them out unless the baby is required to look very fine for a brief display to some friend. These delicate, fancy trifles when once wet through or vomited on are ruined, and it should be your aim to leave everything as good as you found it when you go from the house. There will be plenty of time after you have left, for the fond mamma to spoil all the pretty things, and as she does so she will appreciate more and more your care of them.

XIII
THE VALLEY OF THE SHADOW

I suppose that no nurse deliberately chooses to go to an incurable case, yet most of us who have done private nursing have found ourselves at some time caring for one who slowly, and painfully, creeps nearer day by day to the great End. We have gone perhaps to stay a few weeks, for some acute disease, but symptoms have changed, and instead of recovery, a long, slow decline is to be faced, the nurse feeling she is needed, decides to stay and do what she can for the poor failing body, and so the weeks drag on in the dreadful monotony of that one sick room, until we feel that we have been left out of the real nursing world, that we are stranded with our patient upon an island of pain, that there is no outlook but the one dread Valley, no moving object but the river of Death, and no hope for the life we are guarding. Each week we grow more and more rusty as to our hardly-won surgical technic, more out of touch with those who come and go to one patient after the other, and who not unnaturally count upon so and so many victories over the very enemy who we know will overcome the life we are fighting to save. Yet we realize that all our care will never bring victory, all our skill can but help to smooth the rugged pathway, down which the feet must tread alone. The endless repetition of the same symptoms is wearying, the only possible variation being some new pain, which indicates another stage in the development of the disease. An improvement hardly cheers us, as we know it is but temporary, and maybe followed by an exacerbation of the trouble.

Often the actual nursing calls but for a portion of the day, but that portion is so necessary that the nurse's presence is imperatively demanded. The remainder of the time little is to be done, except perhaps a guard maintained over the failing strength, a watch kept for untoward accidents that might snap the frail thread that binds the spirit still to earth. Probably the bedroom must be kept tidy, and the patient's clothing cared for, and the nurse feels she has degenerated into a servant.

One who has gone through with an experience like this, and who has courageously remained with her patient to the end, has passed through a training more severe than any she has had in her hospital life, and she has earned a new diploma.

There are some things which the nurse may do to lighten these dark days, some things which may help both herself and her patient, and these I will try to show.

Firstly, it is well to study your case from a pathological view point. Find out the heredity, the manner of the daily life, the first manifestation of the disease, what circumstances led to it, how it was treated, what success the treatment seemed to have, what symptoms can now be noted, what complications have shown themselves, and their influence on the original disease. A careful history could be written embracing all of these points, and as new symptoms appear they should be observed and noted. All this should be valuable and should help some future day to show some one who has but started on the dreaded pathway, how to avoid what will surely be a fatal disease. Many a valuable paper could be written in the long hours when the nurse feels she is losing her time, if she would intelligently study her case, and write the story of the disease, what led to it, and how it is being combated.

Perhaps, if it could be arranged, the nurse might be spared part of a day once or twice a week, and she could go to her hospital out patient department, or to some dispensary and do some work that carries a little feeling of success with it; work in a babies milk station, or almost any of the numerous charitable activities, would rest and refresh one who has for months been with the same patient.

Secondly, as a psychological study. We all know we must die, we feel that we talk to people every day who perhaps will not be alive a twelvemonth hence; but we are not actually certain that ourselves or any of our friends will so soon be dead, and we habitually act and speak as if we all were to live on indefinitely. So to be closely associated with some one who we know is drawing closer and closer to the life beyond the grave, is a very solemn thing; whether the sick one knows it or not, the nurse knows it, and such an one must be viewed with peculiar interest.

She is so near to knowing the great Mystery. She will so soon see those who have gone before. The present helplessness will so marvelously become Life Everlasting. It seems, as the end comes nearer, and yet more near, as if, perhaps, one could send a message to some of our own loved ones gone on before, "If you see some of my dear ones, on that other shore, bear them a loving greeting from me, tell them I am trying to live as they would have me live." Such a thought trembles on the tongue, so near does the unseen seem to come to us.

In the face of these things, how small do the thoughts of our own dignity seem. It is all *service*, and service is what we were made for.

"I pass this way but once, if, therefore, there is *any* service I can perform for my fellow man let me do it now, for I shall not pass this way again." This quotation is familiar to all, and especially does it come to mind when we minister to those who are to die. When they are gone there will be no bringing them back to explain duties slighted or left undone. "We pass this way but once."

Thirdly, from a religious point of view. It is quite impossible to say, what exactly is the nurse's duty as regards the religious side of her ministration, though the wish to help must be often in the mind of every thoughtful nurse who has charge of an incurable case.

The patient may not know her condition, and the doctor may not wish her to be told, then, of course, the nurse's lips must be sealed, as to any allusion to the dread truth. The religious views of the patient and her friends may be different from anything that the nurse knows, or perhaps the family pastor comes frequently, and instructs and comforts the sick one, and the family.

A patient will sometimes *ask* for the reading of some portion of the Bible, and unless the part is specified the nurse may be at a loss just where to turn. Some parts of the Scriptures are so generally known and accepted, that they can hardly fail to give hope and comfort, no matter what the religious teaching may have been heretofore.

I will suggest then *in case* readings are asked for. The Psalms are full of beautiful comforting thoughts and prayers. The 23d has helped many a poor soul about to take its last journey, the 37th, which begins "Fret not thyself," shows that those are truly blessed who trust in the Lord, the 51st, "Have mercy upon me, O God," teaches repentance, the 42d, "As the hart pants after the water-brooks, so longeth my soul for Thee, O God," shows the desire of the soul for God.

In the New Testament, the 14th chapter of St. John's gospel is a universal favorite, on account of its comforting thoughts "In my Father's house are many mansions." In St. Luke's gospel chapter 15th, verse 11, we have the parable of the Prodigal Son, to show how complete and perfect is God's love, and His forgiveness, when sin is forsaken. In 1st Corinthians, 15th chapter, verse 20, we have a masterly argument for the resurrection from the dead, and a life beyond the grave. In Revelations, 14th chapter, 13th verse, is a very comforting thought for those who have led a strenuous life and are in much suffering.

These few references will help, I hope, if any nurse is called upon to read the Bible, and she feels a little nonplussed as to exactly where to turn.

There are of course innumerable passages besides these, that could be found by the aid of a concordance, and which it would be wise to note on a slip of paper, ready for any call. Sometimes a patient will ask for a prayer, and it is not often that a nurse would feel competent to kneel down by the bedside and make an acceptable extemporaneous prayer, so I would suggest buying a volume of "Prayers for the Sick."

Very tiny, dainty little books can be purchased at the church book stores, full of these prayers.

In the Episcopal Book of Common Prayer are many helpful prayers.

The sentence, the collect, and the whole of the Easter service in this book are radiant with the truths of the Resurrection, and the Easter hymns are tuned to the same inspiring theme.

This last thought I leave with you. What more helpful consideration can come to a weary nurse, than that the sick one to whom she has ministered for so many weeks or months should at last, on entering in to the life Eternal, lay before the Lord of Glory, the name of the one who was with her, who helped her, who cared for her, and who was faithful to her trust to the end?